Cognitive Behavioral Therapies for Insomnia

Editor

JASON C. ONG

SLEEP MEDICINE CLINICS

www.sleep.theclinics.com

Consulting Editor
TEOFILO LEE-CHIONG Jr

June 2019 • Volume 14 • Number 2

ELSEVIER

1600 John F. Kennedy Boulevard • Suite 1800 • Philadelphia, Pennsylvania, 19103-2899

http://www.theclinics.com

SLEEP MEDICINE CLINICS Volume 14, Number 2
June 2019, ISSN 1556-407X, ISBN-13: 978-0-323-67809-4

Editor: Colleen Dietzler
Developmental Editor: Donald Mumford

Sleep Medicine Clinics (ISSN 1556-407X) is published quarterly by Elsevier Inc., 360 Park Avenue South, New York, NY 10010-1710. Months of issue are March, June, September and December. Business and Editorial Offices: 1600 John F. Kennedy Blvd., Ste. 1800, Philadelphia, PA 19103-2899. Customer Service Office: 3251 Riverport Lane, Maryland Heights, MO 63043. Periodicals postage paid at New York, NY and additional mailing offices. Subscription prices are $212.00 per year (US individuals), $100.00 (US students), $486.00 (US institutions), $264.00 (Canadian individuals), $252.00 (international individuals) $135.00 (Canadian and international students), $551.00 (Canadian institutions) and $551.00 (International institutions). Foreign air speed delivery is included in all *Clinics* subscription prices. All prices are subject to change without notice. **POSTMASTER:** Send change of address to *Sleep Medicine Clinics*, Elsevier Health Sciences Division, Subscription Customer Service, 3251 Riverport Lane, Maryland Heights, MO 63043. Customer Service: **Tel: 1-800-654-2452 (U.S. and Canada); 314-447-8871 (outside U.S. and Canada). Fax: 314-447-8029. E-mail: journalscustomerservice-usa@elsevier.com (for print support); journalsonlinesupport-usa@elsevier.com (for online support).**

Reprints. For copies of 100 or more of articles in this publication, please contact the Commercial Reprints Department, Elsevier Inc., 360 Park Avenue South, New York, NY 10010-1710. Tel.: 212-633-3874; Fax: 212-633-3820; E-mail: reprints@elsevier.com.

Sleep Medicine Clinics is covered in *MEDLINE/PubMed (Index Medicus)*.

SLEEP MEDICINE CLINICS

SERIES OF RELATED INTEREST

Clinics in Chest Medicine
Available at: https://www.chestmed.theclinics.com/

THE CLINICS ARE AVAILABLE ONLINE!
Access your subscription at:
www.theclinics.com

Contributors

CONSULTING EDITOR

TEOFILO LEE-CHIONG Jr, MD
Professor of Medicine, National Jewish Health,
University of Colorado Denver, Denver,
Colorado, USA; Chief Medical Liaison, Philips
Respironics, Pennsylvania, USA

EDITOR

JASON C. ONG, PhD
Associate Professor, Department of
Neurology, Center for Circadian and Sleep
Medicine, Northwestern University Feinberg
School of Medicine, Chicago, Illinois, USA

AUTHORS

SAMINA AHMED-JAUREGUI, PsyD
Clinical Psychologist, Senior Instructor at Case
Western Medical School, Department of
Pulmonology and Sleep Medicine, University
Hospitals, Cleveland, Ohio, USA

JOHN TODD ARNEDT, PhD
Co-Director, Associate Professor of Psychiatry
and Neurology, Sleep and Circadian Research
Laboratory, Department of Psychiatry,
Michigan Medicine, University of Michigan,
Ann Arbor, Michigan, USA

LAUREN D. ASARNOW, PhD
Instructor, Department of Psychiatry and
Behavioral Sciences, Stanford University,
Stanford, California, USA

LUIS F. BUENAVER, PhD
Assistant Professor, Departments of
Psychiatry and Behavioral Sciences, and
Neurology, Johns Hopkins School of Medicine,
Baltimore, Maryland, USA

DANIEL J. BUYSSE, MD
Professor, Sleep and Chronobiology Center,
Department of Psychiatry, University of
Pittsburgh, Pittsburgh, Pennsylvania, USA

JANET M.Y. CHEUNG, PhD
School of Pharmacy, Faculty of Medicine and
Health, The University of Sydney, Sydney,
Australia; École de psychologie, Université
Laval, Centre d'étude des troubles du
sommeil, Institut universitaire en santé
mentale de Québec, Québec, Québec,
Canada

ED DE BRUIN, PhD
Research Institute of Child Development and
Education, University of Amsterdam,
Amsterdam, the Netherlands

JULIA DEWALD-KAUFMANN, PhD
Department of Psychiatry and Psychotherapy,
University Hospital, LMU Munich, Hochschule
Fresenius, University of Applied Sciences,
Munich, Germany

MICHELLE L. DRERUP, PsyD, DBSM
Director of Behavioral Sleep Medicine, Sleep
Disorders Center, Cleveland Clinic, Clinical
Assistant Professor of Medicine, Cleveland
Clinic Lerner College of Medicine, Cleveland,
Ohio, USA

JASON G. ELLIS, PhD
Professor of Sleep Science, Northumbria
Sleep Research Laboratory, Faculty of
Health and Life Sciences, Northumbria
University, Newcastle upon Tyne,
United Kingdom

SHEILA N. GARLAND, PhD
Department of Psychology, Faculty of Science,
Division of Oncology, Faculty of Medicine,
Memorial University of Newfoundland,
St. John's, Newfoundland, Canada

HEATHER E. GUNN, PhD
Assistant Professor, Department of
Psychology, University of Alabama,
Tuscaloosa, Alabama, USA

XIAO-WEN JI, PhD
École de psychologie, Université Laval, Centre
d'étude des troubles du sommeil, Institut
universitaire en santé mentale de Québec,
Québec, Québec, Canada

VICTORIA A.J. KAVANAGH, BA
Department of Psychology, Faculty of
Science, Memorial University of
Newfoundland, St. John's, Newfoundland,
Canada

MONICA R. KELLY, PhD
Geriatric Research, Education and Clinical
Center, VA Greater Los Angeles Healthcare
System, VA Sepulveda Ambulatory
Care Center, North Hills, California,
USA

LEON LACK, PhD
Emeritus Professor, College of Education,
Psychology and Social Work, Flinders
University, Adelaide, South Australia,
Australia

NICOLE LOVATO, PhD
Postdoctoral Fellow, Adelaide Institute for
Sleep Health, College of Medicine and Public
Health, Flinders University, South Australia,
Australia

RACHEL MANBER, PhD
Professor, Department of Psychiatry and
Behavioral Sciences, Stanford University,
Stanford, California, USA

JENNIFER L. MARTIN, PhD
Geriatric Research, Education and Clinical
Center, VA Greater Los Angeles Healthcare
System, VA Sepulveda Ambulatory Care
Center, North Hills, California, USA;
Department of Medicine, David Geffen
School of Medicine, University of California,
Los Angeles, Los Angeles, California,
USA

JESSICA M. MEERS, MA
Department of Psychology, University of
Houston, Houston, Texas, USA

GRADISAR MICHAEL, PhD
School of Psychology, Flinders University,
Adelaide, South Australia

CHARLES M. MORIN, PhD
École de psychologie, Université Laval, Centre
d'étude des troubles du sommeil, Institut
universitaire en santé mentale de Québec,
Québec, Québec, Canada

SARA NOWAKOWSKI, PhD
Assistant Professor, Department of Obstetrics
and Gynecology, University of Texas Medical
Branch, Galveston, Texas, USA

JASON C. ONG, PhD
Associate Professor, Department of
Neurology, Center for Circadian and Sleep
Medicine, Northwestern University Feinberg
School of Medicine, Chicago, Illinois,
USA

GRETA B. RAGLAN, PhD
Sleep and Circadian Research Laboratory,
Department of Psychiatry, Michigan Medicine,
University of Michigan, Ann Arbor, Michigan,
USA

JOSHUA A. RASH, PhD
Department of Psychology, Faculty of
Science, Memorial University of
Newfoundland, St. John's, Newfoundland,
Canada

RUTH ROBBINS, PhD
VA Greater Los Angeles Healthcare System,
Department of Psychology, VA Sepulveda
Ambulatory Care Center, North Hills, California,
USA

HANNAH SCOTT, BPsych (Hons)
PhD student, College of Education,
Psychology and Social Work, Flinders
University, Adelaide, South Australia, Australia

LESLIE M. SWANSON, PhD
Sleep and Circadian Research Laboratory,
Department of Psychiatry, Michigan Medicine,
University of Michigan, Ann Arbor, Michigan, USA

DONALD TOWNSEND, PhD
Associate Professor, Arizona School of
Professional Psychology at Argosy University,
Phoenix, Arizona, USA

JOSHUA TUTEK, MA
Department of Psychology, University
of Alabama, Tuscaloosa, Alabama,
USA

Contents

Section 1: Delivery of CBT-I in Specific Populations

> Insomnia is one of the most prevalent sleep disorders in school-aged children and ad-
> olescents. Although cognitive behavioral therapy for insomnia (CBT-i) is the first-line
> treatment for adults, and existing studies show promising effects also for children
> and adolescents, the number of randomized controlled trials in younger age groups
> is rather small. CBT-i techniques for school-aged children and adolescents include
> bedtime shifts (including sleep restriction), stimulus control, thought challenging, psy-
> choeducation, and relaxation techniques. The integration of parents, especially in
> school-aged children with insomnia, is highly recommended. More research is needed
> to investigate specific characteristics and models of child and adolescent insomnia.

> Insomnia is highly comorbid with other mental health and medical conditions and
> adversely affects quality of life and daytime functioning. Cognitive behavioral ther-
> apy for insomnia (CBT-I) is a safe and efficacious treatment for insomnia in the
> context of various comorbid conditions. In this article, the authors outline consider-
> ations for delivering CBT-I in patients with the most common co-occurring medical
> and mental health conditions, review the evidence for CBT-I in these populations as
> well as special considerations for its application, and highlight future areas for
> research in the area of CBT-I for comorbid medical and psychiatric conditions.

> This article reviews the literature on cognitive behavioral therapy for insomnia in adults
> and adolescents with depression. Recent research has expanded on previous research,
> which established that sleep problems are an important predictor of depression and that
> sleep problems are associated with more severe depression, more suicidality, and
> worse outcomes for treatment of depression. The relationship between sleep problems
> and depression is complex, likely bidirectional, and impactful. To further improve the
> lives of patients with depression who experience insomnia, it will be important to inves-
> tigate which patients will do better in a sequential versus concomitant approach.

> Differences in sleep for men and women begin at a very early age, with women re-
> porting poorer sleep and having a higher risk for insomnia compared with men.

immediately effective and durable treatment of sleep-onset insomnia. Its major disadvantage of dependence on sleep laboratory resources has now been overcome with the development of wearable devices using behavioral responses as the indicator of sleep onset to allow for the inexpensive, practical administration of ISR at home.

Section 3: Considerations and Controversies Related to CBT-I

Preface

Cognitive and Behavioral Therapies for Insomnia: Who Is It for? What's New? Where Do We Go from Here?

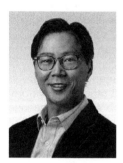

Jason C. Ong, PhD
Editor

Psychological and behavioral treatments have been used to treat insomnia for several decades. The first group of behavioral treatments used relaxation strategies, such as progressive muscle relaxation and biofeedback, to reduce physiologic arousal, which was thought to be the cause of insomnia. During the 1970s and 1980s, theory-driven approaches, including stimulus control,[1] sleep hygiene,[2] and sleep restriction therapy,[3] were developed. As research began to implicate the role of cognitive factors (eg, maladaptive beliefs and attitudes about sleep, high effort to sleep) in chronic insomnia,[4] techniques aimed at the cognitive level emerged. These individual techniques have been combined into a multicomponent treatment package that is known as cognitive behavior therapy for insomnia (CBT-I).

CBT-I is now recognized as the first-line treatment for chronic insomnia disorder.[5] Despite this recognition, some controversies and unresolved questions remain. First, who should receive CBT-I? Is this a one-size-fits-all treatment package, and does it work the same for patients with various comorbid conditions? Second, are there alternatives to CBT-I? What is the evidence for these other nonpharmacologic approaches, and when should they be considered a treatment option? Third, how can we spread CBT-I to the masses? Although CBT-I has demonstrated evidence for efficacy, it remains massively

underutilized relative to the high prevalence of insomnia. What are the barriers, and how do we address this problem?

This issue of *Sleep Medicine Clinics* addresses these questions by providing reviews on several key topics related to cognitive and behavioral treatments for insomnia. The first five articles discuss the delivery of CBT-I to specific populations. Gradisar and colleagues provide an overview of CBT-I in children and adolescents, an area that has received surprisingly little attention. In the next article, Arendt and colleagues discuss considerations in the delivery of CBT-I in patients with comorbid medical and psychiatric conditions, since insomnia often occurs with other conditions. Given the common cooccurrence of insomnia and depression, Arsanow and Manber provide an in-depth review of delivering CBT-I for adolescents and adults with comorbid depression. With emerging interest in sleep and women's health, Nowakoski and Meers provide an overview of CBT-I in women, describing factors associated with pregnancy, menstrual cycles, and menopause. Finally, Martin and colleagues discuss issues in delivering CBT-I to military personnel, who typically present with complex physical and mental issues.

The second section of this issue includes articles on new alternatives or adaptations of CBT-I. Mindfulness meditation is a popular alternative

Sleep Med Clin 14 (2019) xiii–xiv
https://doi.org/10.1016/j.jsmc.2019.02.004
1556-407X/19/© 2019 Published by Elsevier Inc.

approach, and Garland and colleagues provide a review and meta-analysis of the randomized controlled trials conducted in this area. Gunn and colleagues provide an overview of Brief Behavior Therapy, a shorter and more portable version of CBT-I. Intensive Sleep Retraining (ISR) is a novel behavioral approach designed to rapidly decrease sleep onset latency in an intense laboratory protocol. Lack and colleagues describe the history and evidence for ISR and explain how technology is now being used to translate the ISR protocol outside of sleep laboratories.

The third section consists of articles related to controversies and considerations of CBT-I. Morin and colleagues discuss the issues with the use of hypnotics when delivering CBT-I. Although CBT-I is an established treatment for chronic insomnia, the management of acute insomnia has generated controversy. Jason Ellis addresses this interesting question and describes a one-shot approach to treating acute insomnia. Buenaver and colleagues discuss issues involved with delivering CBT-I in the real world, including who is an appropriate candidate, using quality measures, and adaptations of CBT-I. In the final article, Drerup and Ahmed-Jauregui provide an overview of on-line delivery of CBT-I, an exciting area where technology is being leveraged to address the limited accessibility to CBT-I providers.

I would like to thank all of the contributors for their collective expertise in bringing this issue together. I hope that this collection of articles will inform the reader of the state-of-the-science and inspire continued innovations and advances in the treatment of insomnia.

Jason C. Ong, PhD
Department of Neurology
Center for Circadian and Sleep Medicine
Northwestern University
Feinberg School of Medicine
710 North Lake Shore Drive
Room 1004
Chicago, IL 60611, USA

E-mail address:
jason.ong@northwestern.edu

REFERENCES

1. Bootzin RR. Stimulus control treatment for insomnia. Presented at the 80th Annual Convention of the American Psychological Association. Honolulu (HI), August, 1972.
2. Hauri PJ. Current concepts: the sleep disorders. Kalamazoo (MI): The Upjohn Company; 1977.
3. Spielman AJ, Sasky P, Thorpy MJ. Treatment of chronic insomnia by restriction of time in bed. Sleep 1987;10(1):45–56.
4. Morin CM. Insomnia: psychological assessment and management. New York: The Guilford Press; 1993.
5. Qaseem A, Kansagara D, Forciea MA, et al. Clinical Guidelines Committee of the American College of P. Management of chronic insomnia disorder in adults: a clinical practice guideline from the American College of Physicians. Ann Intern Med 2016;165(2):125–33.

Cognitive Behavioral Therapy for Insomnia (CBT-i) in School-Aged Children and Adolescents

Julia Dewald-Kaufmann, PhD[a,b,*], Ed de Bruin, PhD[c],
Gradisar Michael, PhD[d]

KEYWORDS

- Insomnia - Children - Adolescents - Sleep problems
- Cognitive behavioral therapy for insomnia (CBT-i)

KEY POINTS

- Insomnia is a common sleep disorder in school-aged children and adolescents with severe consequences on daytime functioning.
- Diagnostic tools should include clinical interviews, questionnaires, and sleep diaries. Objective sleep assessments (actigraphy, polysomnography) can additionally be used, especially when other sleep disorders (eg, sleep apnea) may be suspected.
- Cognitive behavioral therapy for insomnia (CBT-i) seems to be effective in school-aged children and adolescents; however, only a limited number of randomized controlled trials exist.
- More replication research, especially in clinical settings, is needed to systematically evaluate the effects of CBT-i in children and adolescents.

INTRODUCTION

One of the most prevalent sleep disorders in children and adolescents is "insomnia," which can be briefly described as problems with initiating and/or maintaining sleep with associated daytime consequences. These are typical insomnia symptoms, and when experienced for long enough, and when they interfere with an important area of the young person's life (eg, schooling), then a diagnosis of an insomnia disorder may be warranted. Prevalence rates of insomnia symptoms are high and range up to 30% in children[1–3] and from ~ 40%[4] to 66%[5] in adolescents, whereas prevalence rates for the full insomnia disorder diagnosis vary between ~ 9% and 23%.[4,6–8] Differences in prevalence rates may be explained by differences in assessment methods and definitions of "sleep problems" and "insomnia" (eg, assessment of symptoms or sleep disorders, using different diagnostic classifications).[6,9] If not treated, insomnia symptoms during childhood and adolescence are often persistent and constitute a risk factor for negative daytime consequences, including

Disclosure Statement: G. Michael has a book contract with the Little Brown Book Company on this topic and has received consultancies from the Australian Psychological Society; there are no other conflicts of interest to declare.
[a] Department of Psychiatry and Psychotherapy, University Hospital, LMU Munich, Nussbaumstr. 7, Munich 80336, Germany; [b] Hochschule Fresenius, University of Applied Sciences, Infanteriestr. 11a, Munich 80797, Germany; [c] Research Institute of Child Development and Education, University of Amsterdam, Nieuwe Achtergracht 127, Amsterdam 1018 WS, the Netherlands; [d] School of Psychology, Flinders University, GPO Box 2100, Adelaide 5001, South Australia
* Corresponding author.
E-mail address: Julia.dewald-kaufmann@hs-fresenius.de

cognitive deficits, behavioral problems, school problems, somatic problems, and emotional problems[10–15]. Although an insomnia disorder includes both problems with initiating and/or maintaining sleep, school-aged children and adolescents mostly suffer from problems with initiating sleep. In addition, children often have behavioral difficulties including bedtime resistance and reluctance/refusal to sleep alone.[1,16]

In the second edition of the International Classification of Sleep Disorders-2 (ICSD-2),[17] the diagnosis of Behavioral Insomnia of Childhood (with limit-setting and sleep-onset association type) captured sleep problems of school-aged children and young adolescents quite well. Indeed, many types of insomnia disorders were provided in the ICSD-2. However, with the introduction of the third edition (ICSD-3), most insomnia disorders were removed in favor of a more simplified approach. This meant specific insomnia disorder subtypes and a special pediatric category no longer exists in the ICSD-3, in which simply a distinction is now made between short-term insomnia and chronic insomnia.[18] These 2 diagnoses solely differ on the criteria of frequency (chronic insomnia requires sleeping problems at least 3 times per week) and the time frame criterion of problems lasting for at least 3 months for chronic insomnia. Most children and adolescents who seek treatment experience sleep problems over a longer time period and therefore fulfill the criteria of a chronic insomnia diagnosis. For example, Paine and Gradisar (2011)[16] found that school-aged children with insomnia were experiencing their sleep problem for 5.7 years, indicating an average age of onset at 3.7 years. Although different etiologic adult models[19] and attempts for models in young children exist,[20] no specific model for school-aged children and adolescents has been developed so far, but an interplay of multiple intrinsic and extrinsic factors is assumed to be crucial.

The recommended first-line treatment for insomnia in adults is cognitive behavioral therapy for insomnia (CBT-i),[21,22] which is a nonpharmacologic treatment that aims to change behavioral (eg, sleep hygiene, bedtime routine) and cognitive (eg, modification of thoughts) patterns in order to improve the individual's sleep. Adult studies show that CBT-i has beneficial and clinically meaningful effects on sleep[22–25] and even on cognitive performance.[26] Furthermore, the effects of CBT-i do not have the drawbacks of pharmacotherapy, such as habituation and dependence.[22,27] However, the number of studies systematically evaluating the effects of CBT-i in children and adolescents is relatively small, and so far no consensus statement has been published for these age groups, which may be because there are so few studies with these populations; however, this may change. Meltzer and Mindell (2014)[28] published a systematic review and meta-analysis on sleep treatments in children and adolescents, which showed that 12 of the 16 included studies focused on infants and young children (birth to 5 years), whereas only 4 studies addressed school-aged children. No randomized controlled trial (RCT) with adolescents could be included in their study at that time. Furthermore, out of the 4 studies on school-aged children, only 1 study applied CBT-i explicitly[16] and 1 study used a brief sleep intervention, which included aspects of CBT-i.[29] A more recent systematic review on CBT-i in adolescents included 9 studies investigating the effects of CBT-i in adolescents,[30] with only 1 RCT that applied CBT-i in adolescents with insomnia without a comorbid disorder.[31]

Before considering CBT-i as a treatment option, children and adolescents should be screened, optimally by parent reports and self-reports, and if necessary treated for physical conditions (eg, allergies, breathing problems, chronic illnesses) that can cause sleeping problems. Because it has been shown that improving sleep has beneficial effects on emotional problems (eg, mood, anxiety),[16,32,33] it is recommended to treat insomnia problems even if it cooccurs with other mental disorders. Still, clinicians should keep comorbidity and situational influences in mind and adapt treatment individually, when needed. In children and adolescents with complaints indicating a delayed sleep-wake phase disorder, dim light melatonin onset (DLMO) should also be assessed, because patients may need exogenous melatonin to fall asleep.[34,35] If a circadian rhythm delay is suspected, the authors recommend clinicians to treat this factor before undertaking CBT-i with the following paper contained within this journal.[36] The diagnostic process of insomnia optimally includes screening questionnaires (self-reports and parent reports), a clinical interview, and sleep diaries (**Table 1**).

In this article, the authors first review the evidence for cognitive and behavioral trials for school-aged children and adolescents and then discuss the practical application of these techniques in each of these populations.

COGNITIVE BEHAVIORAL THERAPY FOR INSOMNIA IN SCHOOL-AGED CHILDREN
Empirical Evidence

The age range of school-aged children recruited into clinical trials evaluating CBT-i has ranged between 5 and 13 years of age.[16,45] It is suggested

Table 1
Diagnostic tools used in the diagnostic process of insomnia in school-aged children and adolescents

Assessment Tool	Specification of Assessment
Sleep disorders and sleep disturbances questionnaires[a]	*Sleep Disturbance Scale for Children*[37]: 6.5–15.3 y, parent report *Children's Sleep Habit Questionnaire*[38]: 4–12 y, parent report *Behavioral Evaluation of Disorders of Sleep Scale (BEDS)*[39]: 5–12 y, parent report
Sleepiness questionnaires [a]	*Cleveland Adolescent Sleepiness Questionnaire*[40]: 11–17 y, self-report *Pediatric Daytime Sleepiness Scale (PDSS)*[41]: 11–15 y, self-report
Sleep hygiene	*Adolescent Sleep Hygiene Scale (ASHS)*[42]: 12–18 y, self-report
Clinical interview	Sleep schedule (bedtime, wake time, naps), evening activities (eg, exercise, social media use, TV), bedtime routine, sleeping environment (eg, lighting, temperature, adequate sleep opportunity), nature of sleep problem (eg, initiating and/or maintaining sleep), night time fears, bedtime refusal and/or need for parental presence, sleepiness and daytime impairments that target diagnostic criteria (eg, emotional problems, school performance), safety behaviors (eg, caffeine, alcohol, medication use, etc.), family and social functioning (eg, stress, life events). Information on what measures have already been taken to improve sleep; prior sleep therapies. Information from parents and teachers on daytime functioning can also be helpful. The clinical interview should also be used to screen for other sleep disorders (eg, apnea, narcolepsy) that should be treated differently.
Sleep diaries[b]	Bedtime, sleep onset latency, number and duration of night time awakenings, wake time, sleep duration, naps. Separate assessment for weekdays and weekends are needed, especially for adolescents.
Actigraphy	Objective assessment of bedtime, sleep onset latency, number and duration of night time awakenings, wake time, sleep duration, and naps can provide additional information. Separate assessment for weekdays and weekends are needed. Actigraphy always requires information from sleep diaries.
Polysomnography	Gives information about sleep architecture, sleep quality, and other sleep related characteristics (eg, breathing). Can be considered if other sleep disorders (eg, sleep apnea) are suspected.
Other technologies (eg, apps, Fitbit)	Aim to measure sleep and wake times; however, their reliability and validity for sleep have not been established. These technologies are therefore not advised for sleep assessment.

[a] Further information and a systematically evaluated list of sleep questionnaires can be found in Spruyt and Gozal, 2011.[43]
[b] See for example Carney et al., 2012.[44]

that fewer school-aged children will be able to grasp the concepts and skills needed for complex cognitive therapy skills, yet this is likely to increase from age 7 years.[16] It is also recognized that the upper end of this age range overlaps with early adolescence (denoted by the onset of puberty). For older school-aged children, the evidence is reviewed here based on the facts that (1) these children do not possess a delayed circadian rhythm contributing to their sleep problem and (2) these children's worries are more centered around issues common in younger school-aged children (eg, fears of harm to self or family members, fears of separation from parents).

Besides the relatively high prevalence rates and the effectiveness of CBT-i in adults, only 2 RCTs have been conducted to investigate the effectiveness of CBT-i in school-aged children.[28] In the first study, Paine and Gradisar (2011)[16] had 42 children between 7 and 13 years randomly assigned to receive either 6 sessions of CBT-i or a waiting list control group. Their results indicate positive effects in the CBT-i group for sleep (sleep latency, wake after sleep onset, sleep efficiency) and anxiety. These improvements were maintained at the 1-month and 6-month follow-ups. However, no changes occurred in total sleep time. In 1 other RCT, school-aged children with insomnia were treated with CBT-i: Schlarb and colleagues[45] (2018) implemented CBT-i, consisting of 3 sessions for children and 3 for parents in 112 children (age range 5–11.5 years). Interventions in this study included sleep restriction, stimulus control therapy, sleep hygiene, relaxation, and cognitive therapy. Results from this study show improvements in sleep problems, sleep onset latency, sleep efficiency, and nocturnal awakenings, but, similar to the study by Paine and Gradisar (2011)[16] no changes in total sleep time were found. Improvements persisted also at the 3-, 6-, and 12-month follow-up assessments. In summary, the limited empirical evidence for CBT-i in school-aged children points toward beneficial effects when treating insomnia; however, more controlled intervention studies are needed to further support these findings. Although other studies have applied sleep interventions for school-aged children (for a review see[28]), these studies (1) did not necessarily focus on children diagnosed with (only) insomnia and/or (2) did not use a combination of behavioral and cognitive techniques. Nevertheless, they frequently used the same techniques as those in the reviewed RCTs and likewise found positive effects on sleep.

Practical Application of cognitive behavioral therapy for insomnia in School-Aged Children

Concerning school-aged children's sleep, parents' behavior plays an essential role.[46] Often parents are not aware of their dysfunctional parenting behavior and develop or maintain a child's sleep problem (eg, child refuses to sleep in the absence of the parent). Furthermore, parents can forget to positively reinforce healthy sleep behaviors (eg, child goes to bed independently, child sleeps through the night.). Thus, children with sleeping problems may experience an imbalance of little positive reinforcement of desirable sleep behaviors and yet too much positive reinforcement of undesirable behaviors, which may perpetuate the sleeping problems. Therefore, CBT-i for school-aged children includes both interventions that relate to the parents and interventions that relate to the child.

Children with insomnia often have problems with initiating sleep, which may take the form of long sleep latencies when trying to sleep independently of a parent. This problem can be addressed by faded bedtimes, an intervention in which bedtimes are scheduled at a later time so the child becomes more sleepy when attempting sleep.[47,48] This technique aims to increase children's sleep pressure and consequently decrease sleep onset latencies and is similar to sleep restriction therapy for adolescents and adults.[49] After sleep latencies decrease, bedtimes can gradually be shifted to an earlier time point, where there is a balance between an appropriate amount of time to fall asleep (eg, <20 min) and no daytime consequences. The implementation of a positive routine before the child's bedtime is also considered to have positive effects on children's sleep, because children enter their bed more relaxed. Consequently, a positive association with the sleeping process (here lying in bed) may occur. Furthermore, moving rewarding components (positive activity with the parent) to a daytime activity helps to extinguish its association with sleep.[47] This intervention is similar to stimulus control therapy for adolescents and adults.[50,51] Positive reinforcement also plays a role when it comes to graduated extinction, during which children are gradually exposed to sleeping alone in their bed, while negative reinforcement (reduced anxiety due to parental attendance) is removed and replaced by positive reinforcement (eg, rewards for successful achievements and practices).[16] **Table 2** provides the step-by-step instructions for both, faded bedtimes and graduated extinction.

Because many children suffer from unpleasant, sleep incompatible feelings and thoughts (eg, "*If I do not fall asleep I will fail at school*"), one important cognitive technique is thought challenging. In the first step, the dysfunctional thought is identified and then in the second step, challenged by looking for evidence for and against these thoughts and/or even replacing it with a more functional/helpful thought. **Box 1** presents a clinical example of thought challenging for a 10-year-old patient with insomnia. As mentioned previously, school-aged children are more likely to engage with cognitive therapy techniques as they become older. As a general rule of thumb, these techniques can be used with children aged 7 years and older,[16] but there are also capable 6-year-olds who can elicit and challenge thoughts and likewise 9-year-olds (and even adults) who have difficulty with such techniques.

In addition to these behavioral and cognitive interventions, CBT-i includes psychoeducation, especially on sleep hygiene, which refers to information about sleeping behaviors and the bedtime routine, because it has been shown that children and adolescents with insomnia often suffer from poor sleep hygiene.[52,53] The general sleep hygiene rules, which should be adapted for each age group, are shown in **Box 2**. In addition, it is important to inform children and their parents about various aspects of sleep, including individual differences in sleep need, sleep homeostatic pressure (as a treatment rationale for faded bedtime),

Table 2
Stepwise procedure: faded bedtimes and graduated extinction

Faded Bedtimes	Graduated Extinction

1. Delay the child's bedtime by 15 min and keep this new bedtime consistent for 1 wk.
2. Ensure the child's wake up time is consistent across the 7 d of the wk.
3. Avoid the child napping
4. After 1 wk, if the child's sleep latency is > 20 min, repeat Step 1 above
5. If the child's sleep latency becomes <20 min, keep to this new bedtime.
6. If daytime consequences occur (eg, sleepiness at school), then advance bedtimes by 15 min for 1 wk
7. Continue Step 6 if daytime consequences still occur
8. The goal is to strike the balance between the length of the child's sleep latency and the severity and/or frequency of their daytime consequences
	1. If child is in the parent's bed, move them to a mattress on the floor next to the parent. After practicing this step to a point where the child is experiencing less fear/anxiety, move the mattress near the bedroom door (either inside or outside the bedroom). After this is practiced enough, move the mattress further toward the child's bedroom (eg, a room near the parents' bedroom). When practiced enough, keep gradually moving the mattress closer to the child's bedroom, until they are in their own bed. *Note:* often a family might decide to go from parents' bed, to a room next to the parents' bed, and then straight to the child's bedroom, as it is more convenient.
	2. If a child is in their own bedroom, but needs the parent close by, then the following steps can be taken:
	  a. Parent may be lying down under the covers with the child.
	  b. Parent lies down on top of the covers with the child.
	  c. Parent sits up on top of the covers with the child.
	  d. Parent sits next to the bed, but lays their hand on the child.
	  e. Parent sits next to the bed, but no contact with the child.
	  f. Parent sits near the end of the child's bed or near the bedroom door.
	  g. Parent is outside the bedroom door (eg, sitting on a chair, etc.).
	  h. Parent gets to reclaim their night and do what they want for themselves.

and sleep architecture (ie, cycling from light-to-deep-to-light stages of sleep). Psychoeducation, and especially sleep hygiene rules, should be provided and discussed in detail before the other CBT-i interventions, as understanding the underlying mechanisms may increase motivation and compliance.

COGNITIVE BEHAVIORAL THERAPY FOR INSOMNIA IN ADOLESCENTS
Empirical Evidence

Similar to the research on CBT-i in children, the scientific literature on the effectiveness of CBT-i in adolescents is rare. Given the positive results from the adult literature and the high prevalence rates of insomnia in adolescents, this constitutes a rather surprising finding. In a recent meta-analysis, Blake and colleagues[30] (2017) found 9 studies that used adolescent cognitive behavioral sleep interventions, which included only 4 RCTs, and only 1 of these RCTs included adolescents with an isolated insomnia diagnosis.[31] The other studies that included adolescents with "insomnia symptoms"/"sleep problems" (with or without comorbid conditions),[50,54–57] adolescents with insomnia and a comorbid psychiatric diagnosis,[58] adolescents with delayed sleep phase disorder[59] were pilot studies[54,57,58,60] and/or uncontrolled studies.[50,54,56,57,61] Still, the results from this meta-analysis showed preliminary positive effects for CBT-i in adolescents, which can be seen in increased sleep durations, decreased sleep onset latencies, decreased wake times after sleep onset, and thus improved sleep efficiency. Furthermore, positive effects were found for sleep quality and daytime functioning, including daytime sleepiness and depressive and anxiety symptoms.[62]

Box 1
Thought challenging of a child

Therapist: What worries you about not being able to fall asleep quickly at night?

Child: That I won't get enough sleep and fail my Maths test.

Therapist: So, every night you have a bad sleep, you're likely to fail a test?

Child: Maybe.

Therapist: OK, so what we can do is see how true that thought is by looking at what's happened in the past. How many times have you failed your test?

Child: Once.

Therapist: OK. So earlier, your mum said that you've had a sleep problem for the last 2 years. How many tests have you had in the past 2 years?

Child: Ummm... probably... about 10.

Therapist: So, you have 5 tests each year?

Child: I guess not. Maybe it's like 12 or 13. Maybe 14?

Therapist: OK. But even so. Whilst you've had a sleep problem over the past 2 years, you have failed 1 test out of about 14.

Child: Yeah.

Therapist: So even though you've slept not-so-great, you passed 13 tests out of 14.

Child: Yeah, I guess I have.

Therapist: So what are the chances of passing a test, even if you haven't slept so great?

Child: I guess they are not so bad.

Box 2
Sleep hygiene rules

- A continuous place to sleep (eg, children and adolescents should have their own bed)
- Regular bedtimes: Bedtimes should be roughly the same each day (also on weekends)
- Avoidance of lying in bed for too long (eg, >30 min), waiting to fall asleep
- Sleep supporting environment (eg, cool air temperature, very dim to no light, minimal noise/sound)
- Avoidance of drinks with caffeine
- Reduction of light before bedtimes (including TV, smartphone, computer usage)
- Reduction of stimulating activities before bedtimes
- Adequate physical activity during the day
- No napping throughout the day

---

improvements were also found in symptoms of psychopathology.[33] Using Internet-based CBT-i was shown to be more cost-effective than group therapy,[63] has the advantage to increase availability and access to treatment, and may also be characterized by high acceptability in adolescent populations. One should be aware that using Internet-based CBT-i requires adolescents to use their computer or mobile phone, possibly close to bedtime, which may contradict sleep hygiene advice; however, the effects of electronic media use on sleep are still not fully understood.[64,65]

Practical Application of Cognitive Behavioral Therapy for Insomnia in Adolescents

Before undertaking CBT-i for adolescents, the authors recommend that clinicians first assess for, and treat, any significant delay in their sleep timing (>2 hour difference between weekday vs weekend bedtimes) that may be due to a delayed circadian rhythm. The rationale behind this is that although cognitive and behavioral techniques are likely to reduce the sleep latency of an adolescent with a delayed circadian rhythm, they are unlikely to advance the timing of their sleep onset time (which may be well past midnight). This delayed sleep onset will perpetuate the restricted sleep of the school-attending adolescent and may prove to become a barrier to treatment. By undertaking chronobiological treatments for the delayed sleep timing,[36] this may provide not only an improvement in an adolescent's sleep phase and duration

Focusing on the only RCT to date that included adolescents with an insomnia diagnosis, de Bruin and colleagues[31] (2015) compared CBT-i (provided as online therapy or group therapy) with a waiting list control group in a sample of 116 adolescents (age range: 12–19 years). The intervention lasted for 6 treatment sessions over 6 weeks, as well as a booster session 2 months after the last treatment session. The program included the following components: psychoeducation/sleep hygiene advice, exercise for worry, thought challenging (ie, cognitive therapy), mindfulness-based relaxation, restriction of time in bed, stimulus control, and finally relapse prevention. Compared with the waiting list control group, both treatment groups improved significantly on sleep efficiency, sleep onset latency, wake after sleep onset, and total sleep time.[31] These improvements were maintained up to a 1-year follow-up, and but also some benefits to any secondary insomnia symptoms.[66]

There exists a gray area between more mild symptoms of delayed sleep phase and insomnia, especially in adolescents. The distinction between the 2—even with a DLMO assessment—is not always easy to make and both can be a predisposing or perpetuating factor for the other[66]. Therefore, the predominant complaint should serve as an important factor to decide which to address first, insomnia or delayed sleep phase, or to address both simultaneously. As a principle rule of thumb for the application of CBT-i, clinicians should decide whether there exists behavioral aspects among the symptoms that are addressed by CBT-i (ie, whether the behavioral techniques from CBT-i will address these symptoms, etc.). If the adolescent suffers solely from a biological predisposition for a severe delayed sleep phase, the application of CBT-I as the first line of treatment is not recommended.

Similar to CBT-i for children, thought challenging and sleep hygiene advice (see descriptions discussed earlier) are important for adolescent treatment of insomnia. The application of these techniques does not differ radically from those described for school-aged children. However, stressing the importance to avoid caffeinated beverages and food[67] and interactive electronic media usage[68] is more relevant in this age group. Furthermore, sleep restriction therapy refers to an intervention that directly addresses the main complaint of most adolescents with insomnia problems, namely, difficulty initiating sleep. Similar to the faded bedtimes described earlier, adolescents are asked to restrict their time in bed in order to consolidate sleep and to decrease sleep onset latencies. The new bedtimes should be

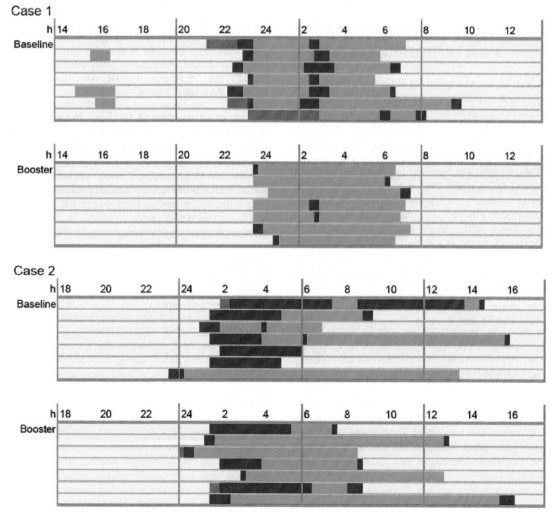

Fig. 1. Sleep diaries of 2 cases (described in **Box 3**) of adolescents with insomnia before and after CBT-i.

determined based on sleep diaries or actigraphy data and have to be discussed with the adolescent.[57] Clinical practice shows that the restriction of time in bed involves going to bed later, as the predominant complaint in adolescent insomnia concerns problems falling asleep, but in some cases the adolescent may prefer to (also) get up earlier. It is important to involve the adolescent in this process, because their agreement to the protocol is needed in order to ensure compliance. This is essential because clinical practice shows that adolescents often experience sleep restriction as a challenging therapeutic technique. Furthermore, it is important to tailor bedtimes to daytime requirements (eg, school) and change the sleeping habits the adolescent has adopted (eg, long naps or a behaviorally shifted circadian rhythm). It is generally advised to restrict sleep until a sleep efficiency (time in bed/total sleep time*100) of 85% to 90% is reached (depended on other personal and lifestyle factors such as age, school start times, leisure activities etc.) and then extending bedtimes gradually (eg, by approximately 15 minutes earlier each week).[57,69,70] Sleep restriction should be repeated immediately when sleep efficiency decreases to 80%. **Fig. 1** demonstrates sleep restriction for 2 clinical cases, highlighting the need to (1) adapt the protocol to the individual, (2) define treatment success differently, and (3) to take other comorbidities for further treatment into account (**Box 3**).

Stimulus control therapy aims to disassociate dysfunctional associations between the bed and waking activity/alertness and instead strengthen the association with sleep.[51] Therefore, adolescents are advised to avoid stimuli that are associated with wakefulness in bed (eg, doing homework on or in the bed) and to avoid going to bed before feeling sleepy. If sleep onset does not occur after 20 to 30 minutes, adolescents are asked to get up for about 15 to 20 minutes and stay awake until they feel sleepy, before going to bed again.[69,71] This process is repeated as long as needed to fall asleep within 20 to 30 minutes.[69] However, if the bedtimes from the sleep restriction therapy exercise are set properly, and going to bed during the forbidden zone of the circadian phase (ie, peak 24-hour circadian alertness) is avoided,[72] stimulus control therapy is rarely needed. In addition, it has been shown that behavioral relaxation techniques (eg, body scan) can reduce sleep onset latencies, whereas the cognitive technique of constructive worry (writing down worries and solutions instead of worrying in bed) does not, because relaxation decreases psychophysiologic arousal when being applied before bedtime.[73]

Box 3
Two cases of adolescents treated with cognitive behavior therapy for insomnia (CBT-i)

Case 1 was a 17-year-old girl with a history of abuse, who lived independently. She had a predominant complaint of waking after sleep onset and short total sleep time. In the top graph it is clearly visible that at baseline she sometimes napped during the day and that her bedtime rhythm was somewhat disrupted. Her total sleep time was approximately 6:00 hours and her sleep efficiency 79%. In the bottom graph, 2 months after CBT-i, her bedtimes had become more regular, and she refrained from napping during the day. Total sleep time had increased to 6:50 hours and sleep efficiency to 95%.

Case 2 was a 14-year-old boy with anxiety problems, who lived alone with his mother. The top graph shows a severe disruption of regular bedtime routines, with long sleep onset latencies and some nights with no sleep at all. The predominant problem seemed to be the absence of daytime routines, which was compounded by the exemption from school for most days because of complex family problems and the infrequent (bedtimes-)support from his mother because of her work hours. At baseline total sleep time was approximately 5:10 hours and sleep efficiency 46%. At 2 months after CBT-i these increased to 7:20 hours and 72%, respectively.

Although both cases showed significant improvements, they also show that after CBT-i there could be residual sleep problems and that sleep problems of adolescents are often strongly influenced by the context, such as parents, family, and school.

SUMMARY

Insomnia is one of the most prevalent sleep disorders in school-aged children and adolescents. Although CBT-i is the first-line treatment for adults, and existing studies show promising effects also for children and adolescents, the number of RCTs in these younger age groups is rather small. CBT-i techniques for school-aged children and adolescents include bedtime shifts (including sleep restriction), stimulus control, thought challenging, psychoeducation about sleep, sleep hygiene, and relaxation techniques. The inclusion of parents, especially in school-aged children with insomnia, is highly recommended. The authors strongly urge the scientific community to conduct further controlled trials, including dismantling trials that evaluate the relative effectiveness of individual CBT-i components (eg, thought challenging, sleep restriction therapy, etc.)[74]; so clinicians can be more confident in using these techniques to better the sleep health of young people. Furthermore, more research is needed to investigate specific characteristics and models of child and adolescent insomnia.

REFERENCES

1. Blader JC, Koplewicz HS, Abikoff H, et al. Sleep problems of elementary school children. A community survey. Arch Pediatr Adolesc Med 1997;151: 473–80.
2. Liu X, Liu L, Owens JA, et al. Sleep patterns and sleep problems among schoolchildren in the United States and China. Pediatrics 2005;115:241–9.
3. Spruyt K, O'Brien LM, Cluydts R, et al. Odds, prevalence and predictors of sleep problems in school-age normal children. J Sleep Res 2005;14:163–76.
4. Chung KF, Kan KKK, Yeung WF. Insomnia in adolescents: prevalence, help-seeking behaviors, and types of interventions. Child and Adolescent Mental Health 2014;19:57–63.
5. Short MA, Gradisar M, Gill J, et al. Identifying adolescent sleep problems. PLoS One 2013;8: e75301.
6. Hysing M, Pallesen S, Stormark KM, et al. Sleep patterns and insomnia among adolescents: a population-based study. J Sleep Res 2013;22:549–56.
7. Johnson EO, Roth T, Schultz L, et al. Epidemiology of DSM-IV insomnia in adolescence: lifetime prevalence, chronicity, and an emergent gender difference. Pediatrics 2006;117:e247–56.
8. Ohayon MM, Roberts RE. Comparability of sleep disorders diagnoses using DSM-IV and ICSD classifications with adolescents. Sleep 2001;24:920–5.
9. Dohnt H, Gradisar M, Short MA. Insomnia and its symptoms in adolescents: comparing DSM-IV and ICSD-II diagnostic criteria. J Clin Sleep Med 2012; 8:295–9.
10. Gregory AM, Sadeh A. Sleep, emotional and behavioral difficulties in children and adolescents. Sleep Med Rev 2012;16:129–36.
11. Beebe DW. Cognitive, behavioral, and functional consequences of inadequate sleep in children and adolescents. Pediatr Clin North Am 2011;58:649–65.
12. Roberts RE, Roberts CR, Chen IG. Impact of insomnia on future functioning of adolescents. J Psychosom Res 2002;53:561–9.
13. Dewald JF, Meijer AM, Oort FJ, et al. The influence of sleep quality, sleep duration and sleepiness on school performance in children and adolescents: a meta-analytic review. Sleep Med Rev 2010;14: 179–89.
14. Shochat T, Cohen-Zion M, Tzischinsky O. Functional consequences of inadequate sleep in adolescents: a systematic review. Sleep Med Rev 2014;18:75–87.
15. Simola P, Liukkonen K, Pitkaranta A, et al. Psychosocial and somatic outcomes of sleep problems in children: a 4-year follow-up study. Child Care Health Dev 2014;40:60–7.
16. Paine S, Gradisar M. A randomised controlled trial of cognitive-behaviour therapy for behavioural insomnia of childhood in school-aged children. Behav Res Ther 2011;49:379–88.
17. American Academy of Sleep Medicine. The international classification of sleep disorders, 2nd edition: diagnostic and coding manual. Westchester (IL): American Academy of Sleep Medicine; 2005.
18. American Academy of Sleep Medicine. The international classification of sleep disorders, 3nd edition: diagnostic and coding manual. Westchester (IL): American Academy of Sleep Medicine; 2014.
19. Perlis M, Shaw PJ, Cano G, et al. Models of insomnia. Principles and practice of sleep medicine 2011;5:850–65.
20. Sadeh R, Anders TF. Infant sleep problems: origins, assessment, Infant Mental Health Journal 1993;14: 17–34.
21. Morgenthaler T, Kramer M, Alessi C, et al. Practice parameters for the psychological and behavioral treatment of insomnia: an update. An american academy of sleep medicine report. Sleep 2006;29: 1415–9.
22. Mitchell MD, Gehrman P, Perlis M, et al. Comparative effectiveness of cognitive behavioral therapy for insomnia: a systematic review. BMC Fam Pract 2012;13:40.
23. Koffel EA, Koffel JB, Gehrman PR. A meta-analysis of group cognitive behavioral therapy for insomnia. Sleep Med Rev 2015;19:6–16.
24. Okajima I, Inoue Y. Efficacy of cognitive behavioral therapy for comorbid insomnia: a meta-analysis. Sleep and Biological Rhythms 2018;16(1):21–35.
25. Trauer JM, Qian MY, Doyle JS, et al. Cognitive behavioral therapy for chronic insomnia: a systematic review and meta-analysis. Ann Intern Med 2015;163:191–204.
26. Herbert V, Kyle SD, Pratt D. Does cognitive behavioural therapy for insomnia improve cognitive performance? A systematic review and narrative synthesis. Sleep Med Rev 2018;39:37–51.
27. Riemann D, Perlis ML. The treatments of chronic insomnia: a review of benzodiazepine receptor agonists and psychological and behavioral therapies. Sleep Med Rev 2009;13:205–14.
28. Meltzer LJ, Mindell JA. Systematic review and meta-analysis of behavioral interventions for pediatric insomnia. J Pediatr Psychol 2014;39:932–48.
29. Quach J, Hiscock H, Ukoumunne OC, et al. A brief sleep intervention improves outcomes in the school entry year: a randomized controlled trial. Pediatrics 2011;128:692–701.

30. Blake MJ, Sheeber LB, Youssef GJ, et al. Systematic review and meta-analysis of adolescent cognitive-behavioral sleep interventions. Clin Child Fam Psychol Rev 2017;20:227–49.

31. de Bruin EJ, Bogels SM, Oort FJ, et al. Efficacy of cognitive behavioral therapy for insomnia in adolescents: a randomized controlled trial with internet therapy, group therapy and a waiting list condition. Sleep 2015;38:1913–26.

32. Blake MJ, Snoep L, Raniti M, et al. A cognitive-behavioral and mindfulness-based group sleep intervention improves behavior problems in at-risk adolescents by improving perceived sleep quality. Behav Res Ther 2017;99:147–56.

33. de Bruin EJ, Bogels SM, Oort FJ, et al. Improvements of adolescent psychopathology after insomnia treatment: results from a randomized controlled trial over 1 year. J Child Psychol Psychiatry 2018;59:509–22.

34. Smits MG, van Stel HF, van der Heijden K, et al. Melatonin improves health status and sleep in children with idiopathic chronic sleep-onset insomnia: a randomized placebo-controlled trial. J Am Acad Child Adolesc Psychiatry 2003;42:1286–93.

35. van Maanen A, Meijer AM, Smits MG, et al. Effects of melatonin and bright light treatment in childhood chronic sleep onset insomnia with late melatonin onset: a randomized controlled study. Sleep 2017;40.

36. Gradisar M, Smits M, Bjorvatn B. Assessment and treatment of delayed sleep phase disorder in adolescents: recent innovations and cautions. Sleep Med Clin 2014;9:199–210.

37. Bruni O, Ottaviano S, Guidetti V, et al. The sleep disturbance scale for children (sdsc). Construction and validation of an instrument to evaluate sleep disturbances in childhood and adolescence. J Sleep Res 1996;5:251–61.

38. Owens JA, Spirito A, McGuinn M. The children's sleep habits questionnaire (cshq): psychometric properties of a survey instrument for school-aged children. Sleep 2000;23:1043–51.

39. Schreck KA, Mulick JA, Rojahn J. Development of the behavioral evaluation of disorders of sleep scale. J Child Fam Stud 2003;12:349–59.

40. Spilsbury JC, Drotar D, Rosen CL, et al. The cleveland adolescent sleepiness questionnaire: a new measure to assess excessive daytime sleepiness in adolescents. J Clin Sleep Med 2007;3:603–12.

41. Drake C, Nickel C, Burduvali E, et al. The pediatric daytime sleepiness scale (pdss): sleep habits and school outcomes in middle-school children. Sleep 2003;26:455–8.

42. LeBourgeois MK, Giannotti F, Cortesi F, et al. The relationship between reported sleep quality and sleep hygiene in Italian and american adolescents. Pediatrics 2005;115:257–65.

43. Spruyt K, Gozal D. Pediatric sleep questionnaires as diagnostic or epidemiological tools: a review of currently available instruments. Sleep Med Rev 2011;15:19–32.

44. Carney CE, Buysse DJ, Ancoli-Israel S, et al. The consensus sleep diary: standardizing prospective sleep self-monitoring. Sleep 2012;35:287–302.

45. Schlarb AA, Bihlmaier I, Velten-Schurian K, et al. Short- and long-term effects of cbt-i in groups for school-age children suffering from chronic insomnia: the kiss-program. Behav Sleep Med 2018;16:380–97.

46. Moore M. Behavioral sleep problems in children and adolescents. J Clin Psychol Med Settings 2012;19:77–83.

47. Kuhn BR, Elliott AJ. Treatment efficacy in behavioral pediatric sleep medicine. J Psychosom Res 2003;54:587–97.

48. Sadeh A. Cognitive-behavioral treatment for childhood sleep disorders. Clin Psychol Rev 2005;25:612–28.

49. Miller CB, Espie CA, Epstein DR, et al. The evidence base of sleep restriction therapy for treating insomnia disorder. Sleep Med Rev 2014;18:415–24.

50. Bootzin RR, Stevens SJ. Adolescents, substance abuse, and the treatment of insomnia and daytime sleepiness. Clin Psychol Rev 2005;25:629–44.

51. Bootzin RR, Perlis ML. Stimulus control therapy. In: Perlis M, Aloia M, Kuhn B, editors. Stimulus control therapy. Behavioral treatments for sleep disorders. New York: Academic Press; 2011. p. 21–30.

52. de Bruin EJ, van Kampen RK, van Kooten T, et al. Psychometric properties and clinical relevance of the adolescent sleep hygiene scale in Dutch adolescents. Sleep Med 2014;15:789–97.

53. Mindell JA, Meltzer LJ, Carskadon MA, et al. Developmental aspects of sleep hygiene: findings from the 2004 national sleep foundation sleep in America poll. Sleep Med 2009;10:771–9.

54. Bei B, Byrne ML, Ivens C, et al. Pilot study of a mindfulness-based, multi-component, in-school group sleep intervention in adolescent girls. Early Interv Psychiatry 2013;7:213–20.

55. Blake M, Waloszek JM, Schwartz O, et al. The sense study: post intervention effects of a randomized controlled trial of a cognitive-behavioral and mindfulness-based group sleep improvement intervention among at-risk adolescents. J Consult Clin Psychol 2016;84:1039–51.

56. Britton WB, Bootzin RR, Cousins JC, et al. The contribution of mindfulness practice to a multicomponent behavioral sleep intervention following substance abuse treatment in adolescents: a treatment-development study. Subst Abus 2010;31:86–97.

57. de Bruin EJ, Oort FJ, Bogels SM, et al. Efficacy of internet and group-administered cognitive

behavioral therapy for insomnia in adolescents: a pilot study. Behav Sleep Med 2014;12:235–54.

58. Clarke G, McGlinchey EL, Hein K, et al. Cognitive-behavioral treatment of insomnia and depression in adolescents: a pilot randomized trial. Behav Res Ther 2015;69:111–8.

59. Gradisar M, Dohnt H, Gardner G, et al. A randomized controlled trial of cognitive-behavior therapy plus bright light therapy for adolescent delayed sleep phase disorder. Sleep 2011;34: 1671–80.

60. Schlarb AA, Liddle CC, Hautzinger M. Just - a multimodal program for treatment of insomnia in adolescents: a pilot study. Nat Sci Sleep 2011;3:13–20.

61. Roeser K, Schwerdtle B, Kübler A, et al. Further evidence for the just program as treatment for insomnia in adolescents: results from a 1-year follow-up study. J Clin Sleep Med 2016;12:257–62.

62. Blake MJ, Blake LM, Schwartz O, et al. Who benefits from adolescent sleep interventions? Moderators of treatment efficacy in a randomized controlled trial of a cognitive-behavioral and mindfulness-based group sleep intervention for at-risk adolescents. J Child Psychol Psychiatry 2018;59:637–49.

63. De Bruin EJ, van Steensel FJ, Meijer AM. Cost-effectiveness of group and internet cognitive behavioral therapy for insomnia in adolescents: results from a randomized controlled trial. Sleep 2016;39:1571–81.

64. Bartel K, Scheeren R, Gradisar M. Altering adolescents' pre-bedtime phone use to achieve better sleep health. Health Commun 2018. [Epub ahead of print].

65. Harris A, Gundersen H, Mork-Andreassen P, et al. Restricted use of electronic media, sleep, performance, and mood in high school athletes–a randomized trial. Sleep Health 2015;1:314–21.

66. Richardson C, Micic G, Cain N, et al. Cognitive "insomnia" processes in delayed sleep-wake phase disorder: do they exist and are they responsive to chronobiological treatment? J Consult Clin Psychol 2018. https://doi.org/10.1037/ccp0000357.

67. Bonnar D, Gradisar M. Caffeine and sleep in adolescents: a systematic review. J Caffeine Res 2015;5: 105–14.

68. Hale L, Kirschen GW, LeBourgeois MK, et al. Youth screen media habits and sleep: sleep-friendly screen behavior recommendations for clinicians, educators, and parents. Child Adolesc Psychiatr Clin N Am 2018;27:229–45.

69. Palermo TM, Bromberg MH, Beals-Erickson S, et al. Development and initial feasibility testing of brief cognitive-behavioral therapy for insomnia in adolescents with comorbid conditions. Clin Pract Pediatr Psychol 2016;4:214–26.

70. Schutte-Rodin S, Broch L, Buysse D, et al. Clinical guideline for the evaluation and management of chronic insomnia in adults. J Clin Sleep Med 2008; 4:487–504.

71. De Bruin EJ, Watermann D, Meijer AM. Slimslapen: cognitieve gedragstherapie voor insomnia (cgt-i) bij adolescenten. In: Breat C, Bögels S, editors. Slimslapen: cognitieve gedragstherapie voor insomnia (cgt-i) bij adolescenten. Protocollaire behandeling voor kinderen en adolescenten met psychische klachten, deel 2. Amsterdam (the Netherlands): Boom; 2013. p. 277–312.

72. Lack LC, Lushington K. The rhythms of human sleep propensity and core body temperature. J Sleep Res 1996;5:1–11.

73. Bartel K, Huang C, Maddock B, et al. Brief school-based interventions to assist adolescents' sleep-onset latency: comparing mindfulness and constructive worry versus controls. J Sleep Res 2018;27:e12668.

74. Gradisar M, Richardson C. Cbt-i cannot rest until the sleepy teen can. Sleep 2015;38:1841–2.

Cognitive Behavioral Therapy for Insomnia in Patients with Medical and Psychiatric Comorbidities

Greta B. Raglan, PhD, Leslie M. Swanson, PhD,
John Todd Arnedt, PhD*

KEYWORDS

- Comorbid • Depression • Diagnosis • Disorder • Insomnia • Comorbidity
- Cognitive behavioral therapy for insomnia (CBT-I)

KEY POINTS

- Insomnia is frequently comorbid with other medical or mental health diagnoses.
- Cognitive behavioral therapy for insomnia (CBT-I) is a safe and effective treatment for insomnia in the context of various comorbid conditions.
- Although CBT-I has been shown to improve symptoms of some comorbid conditions, gains are typically stronger in sleep symptoms.
- Some comorbid conditions require modifications or special considerations when enacting components of CBT-I.
- Future research is needed to better establish the effectiveness of CBT-I in patients with comorbid conditions, as well as research on treatment sequencing and alternative methods of CBT-I delivery.

INTRODUCTION

Insomnia is a highly common condition that affects individuals across the lifespan. Up to 20% of Americans report insomnia symptoms[1] and about 9% report symptoms consistent with a clinical diagnosis of insomnia.[2] Most of the patients who experience insomnia do so in the context of comorbid medical or psychiatric conditions[3]; indeed, up to a quarter of individuals with insomnia have comorbid psychiatric conditions,[4] and estimates of insomnia comorbid with medical illness range from 16% to 82%.[5]

Cognitive behavioral therapy for insomnia (CBT-I) is a well-validated, effective, and safe intervention for primary insomnia, and an emerging body of work has demonstrated its efficacy in treating comorbid insomnia. Improvements with CBT-I treatment are observed, for instance, in nonsleep symptoms related to depression,[6] bipolar disorder, posttraumatic stress disorder (PTSD), generalized anxiety disorder (GAD), and chronic pain. Other studies have demonstrated improvement in quality of life, even without change in the comorbid condition (eg, cancer and chronic pain). In general, CBT-I has been used adjunctively to the treatment of a comorbid illness, but recent studies have also tested CBT-I as a monotherapy with the aim of improving both sleep and the comorbid condition. Findings to date suggest that, when used as a monotherapy, CBT-I improves sleep more than symptoms of comorbid conditions.[7] In this article, the authors review general considerations for delivering CBT-I in patients with specific medical and psychiatric conditions that often co-occur with insomnia, discuss the evidence for CBT-I in these populations along

Disclosures Statement: The authors have no relevant financial disclosures.
Sleep and Circadian Research Laboratory, Department of Psychiatry, Michigan Medicine, University of Michigan, 4250 Plymouth Road, Ann Arbor, MI 48109-2700, USA
* Corresponding author.
E-mail address: tarnedt@med.umich.edu

with special considerations for each population, and explore implications for future directions.

TREATMENT SEQUENCING AND CLINICAL CONTRAINDICATIONS

Although CBT-I has fewer contraindications than pharmacologic treatment for insomnia, many of the contraindications involve comorbid illnesses. CBT-I is generally contraindicated in patients with unstable comorbid illnesses that might either directly adversely affect sleep and/or affect the patient's ability to engage in therapy fully.[8] For instance, an individual experiencing an active manic episode or who is actively misusing alcohol would not benefit from CBT-I until these states have resolved.

Patient treatment preference is often an underappreciated variable in the treatment process but can significantly affect treatment outcome. In general, patients with chronic insomnia should be advised of the benefits and risks associated with both pharmacologic and nonpharmacologic evidence-based insomnia treatments and choose the treatment approach that best suits their individual circumstances.

Some comorbid conditions, such as epilepsy, bipolar disorder, active cancer treatment, pregnancy, or chronic pain, may require modifications to CBT-I. For example, time in bed restriction, a component of CBT-I, may be unsafe for individuals with seizure disorders. Similarly, sleep restriction may increase the risk of mania or hypomania among patients with bipolar disorder. Modifications to sleep restriction, such as sleep compression,[9] may be a viable alternative in these circumstances. Modifications and sequencing adjustments for specific comorbid conditions will be discussed later in further detail. A general algorithm for treatment indications can be found in **Fig. 1**.

COMORBID PSYCHIATRIC CONDITIONS
Mood Disorders

Depression
Insomnia and hypersomnolence are diagnostic features of depression. About 40% of individuals with depression also meet criteria for a diagnosis of insomnia and the majority experiences some symptoms of insomnia or sleep disturbance.[3] Symptoms of both depression and insomnia are improved following CBT-I,[6,10,11] and CBT-I seems to be effective even among individuals with more severe depressive symptoms.[10] In addition, electronically delivered CBT-I is effective in improving sleep as well as reducing severity of depression symptoms.[12–14] Depression symptoms, however,

can lead to higher rates of dropout[15] and those with more severe symptoms may be less adherent to treatment recommendations.[10] Sequencing of treatment is therefore an important consideration in this population to ascertain whether to focus first on symptoms of insomnia or depression, or to attempt concurrent treatment. For instance, if a patient's primary depression symptoms involve amotivation, treatment for depression might be prioritized initially in order to build the patient's capacity to engage in CBT-I.

Bipolar disorder
Sleep is particularly important for individuals with bipolar disorder, because sleep loss may result in mood disruption. Poor sleep is prevalent among this population; up to 55% of individuals with bipolar disorder may experience insomnia symptoms even during euthymic periods.[16] Treating insomnia in bipolar patients improves sleep outcomes, such as reduced insomnia severity and higher rates of insomnia remission, as well as preventing relapse of mood episodes over time,[17] indicating that it is an effective tool for improving disease burden and functioning. Because mania or hypomania may affect treatment and adherence, close monitoring for symptoms of mania is important. Sleep restriction has been historically contraindicated in bipolar patients due to the possibility of triggering mania or hypomania; however, recent evidence suggests that, with close monitoring, sleep restriction may be used in patients with bipolar disorder without triggering significant mood changes.[18] While engaging in CBT-I with patients who have bipolar disorder, it is important to set consistent sleep and wake times and regularly monitor total sleep time, sleepiness, and mood for significant changes that might indicate a shift toward mania. More specialized sleep diaries, specific to patients with bipolar, may also help to better characterize the unique symptom presentation of this population.[17]

Perinatal mood disorders
Sleep problems are common during the perinatal period,[19] and insomnia is a significant predictor of poor mood outcomes for pregnant and postpartum women.[20] Sleep may be particularly disrupted during this time by physiologic changes caused by pregnancy and childbirth and the demands of caring for an infant. In a recent survey of treatment preferences, pregnant women indicated a preference for CBT-I over other available treatments for insomnia, such as pharmacotherapy.[21] At least one study has demonstrated the effectiveness of CBT-I in pregnancy[22] and one has shown promise among postpartum women with depression.[23] However, to date, no

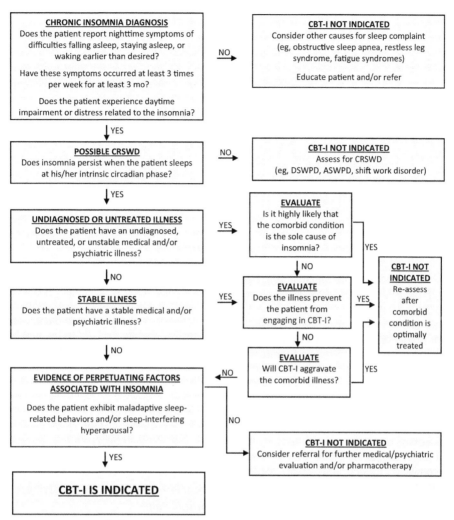

Fig. 1. Decision-to-treat comorbid insomnia algorithm: Is CBT-I indicated? ASWPD, advanced sleep-wake phase disorder; CRSWD, circadian rhythm sleep-wake disorder; DSWPD, delayed sleep-wake phase disorder. (*Adapted from* Smith MT, Perlis ML. Who is a candidate for cognitive-behavioral therapy for insomnia? Health Psychol 2006;25(1):17; with permission.)

randomized controlled trials exist, and further study is warranted.

Because of physiologic changes experienced during pregnancy and in the postpartum period, the requirement for stimulus control (ie, leaving bed when awake) may be relaxed for patients. In these cases, women may engage in relaxing, quiet activities in bed when awake as long as they are not trying to fall asleep (so-called countercontrol). Postpartum women may also be encouraged to breastfeed in bed if that is where they feel most comfortable doing so. Postpartum women should be educated about the adverse effects of light exposure on symptoms of insomnia and should use low lighting whenever possible during nighttime infant care.

Substance Use Disorders

Insomnia and sleep disturbance is common among individuals with alcohol use disorders, with some estimates as high as 90% for sleep disturbances in treatment-seeking adults with alcohol use disorders.[24] Although CBT-I is an effective treatment for insomnia in individuals with alcohol use disorder, two randomized controlled trials did not demonstrate improvements in alcohol use,[25,26] whereas a more recent Ukrainian study found benefits for both sleep (as measured by the Sleep Problems Questionnaire) and alcohol use.[27] Although the findings regarding the relationship between sleep and relapse are mixed to date, there is evidence that sleep difficulties often precede relapse.[28] Future adequately powered trials are needed to determine whether insomnia treatment improves relapse and other aspects of daytime functioning that might facilitate improved recovery.

An important consideration for treating insomnia in the context of alcohol use disorders is ongoing monitoring of use and assessment for intoxication when warranted.[29] Because alcohol can directly disrupt sleep patterns, an emphasis on abstinence during CBT-I is recommended. Abstinence, however, does not guarantee an immediate return to normal sleep patterns, and alcohol-related sleep problems typically persist for months to years after abstinence is achieved.[28,30] No definitive timeline has been determined for the ideal length of abstinence before engaging in CBT-I; however, a common practice is to wait at least one month before initiating CBT-I to allow for any adverse sleep effects related directly to alcohol withdrawal to subside.

In cannabis use disorder, poor sleep quality is an important predictor of a person's likelihood of relapsing during treatment.[31] Sleep is therefore a central area of focus for intervention in order to improve treatment outcomes for this population. Indeed, at least one pilot study has demonstrated that app-delivered CBT-I improves sleep quality among veterans with cannabis use disorder as well as reducing cannabis use, even in the absence of other substance use treatments.[32] Although promising, further large-scale studies are needed in this population.

Anxiety Disorders

Posttraumatic stress disorder
There is significant overlap between PTSD and insomnia. Indeed, about 70% of individuals experiencing PTSD may also experience symptoms of insomnia.[33] Importantly, treatment for PTSD alone does not typically resolve insomnia symptoms.[34] However, CBT-I may improve PTSD symptoms, including nightmares[35] and fear of sleep,[36] as well as reducing alcohol use in patients with PTSD.[37] It has also been shown to improve overall quality of life in patients with PTSD.[35] Patients who are actively undergoing exposure therapy should not receive concurrent CBT-I[38] due to the possibility that PTSD symptoms (eg, nightmares, hyperarousal, aversion to silence) elicited during exposure therapy may interfere with CBT-I engagement. Treatment for PTSD symptoms before CBT-I may be the most effective sequence and, as with all therapeutic interventions, symptoms must be carefully monitored to ensure that care is not compromised.[38]

Generalized anxiety disorder
Individuals with GAD are more likely to experience insomnia, and GAD patients with insomnia have worse outcomes than those without.[39] The important role of anxious ruminations in maintaining insomnia is likely related to these findings. Effective in reducing insomnia severity in this population, CBT-I may also reduce anxiety symptoms as measured by the State-Trait Anxiety Index.[11] CBT-I may be a particularly useful intervention for individuals with comorbid anxiety because many skills emphasized in CBT-I (eg, cognitive restructuring, relaxation, constructive worry) directly target anxiety. At least one study, however, has shown that CBT-I is more effective when GAD is treated before the implementation of CBT-I.[40]

Conclusions
Overall, the body of available evidence suggests that CBT-I is effective in treating insomnia in the context of comorbid psychiatric conditions.[41] Indeed, it has been shown to be as effective in individuals with comorbid psychiatric conditions as in those with primary insomnia.[42] Further, recent work has shown the value of CBT-I for addressing comorbid symptoms, including reduced risk of relapse in bipolar disorder, improvements in substance use in alcohol and cannabis use disorders, and improved quality of life in patients with depression.

COMORBID MEDICAL CONDITIONS
Chronic Pain

At least 50% of patients with chronic pain also experience disturbed sleep, although some estimates are even higher.[43] At least one study has shown additional improvements in self-reported pain among patients with fibromyalgia, although this was a relatively modest change in a small sample.[44] Most studies of the efficacy of CBT-I in treating patients with chronic pain have shown improvement in sleep symptoms, but few demonstrable impacts on self-reported pain.[45–48] Most studies have shown an overall improvement in well-being and quality of life, such as reduced disability and fatigue, even in the absence of direct changes to pain.[48]

Patients with chronic pain may report difficulty in getting out of bed when they are unable to sleep due to pain, frailty, or the use of pain medications. Thus, countercontrol strategies may be preferred to stimulus control guidelines for many of these patients. Alternatives to progressive muscle relaxation exercises may also need to be considered, because this exercise may lead to pain or spasms; alternatively, patients can be instructed to avoid tensing muscles too much.[38]

Perimenopause

Perimenopause marks an approximately 20% increase in sleep disturbance in women,[49] and more than a quarter of women may experience some degree of insomnia during perimenopause.[50,51] Perimenopausal women are also at an increased risk of depression and may be at increased risk for sleep-disordered breathing,[52] which can both contribute to poor sleep. Vasomotor symptoms have been tied to disrupted sleep patterns in perimenopausal women, which may contribute to the presence of insomnia.[53] During perimenopause, CBT-I outperforms many pharmacologic and nonpharmacologic treatments of insomnia.[54] Further, telephone delivery of CBT-I was found to be effective in this population.[55] Although CBT-I has not been shown to directly improve vasomotor symptoms associated with perimenopause, McCurry and colleagues[55] demonstrated than telephone delivery of CBT-I was associated with a reduction in reported sleep disruption caused by vasomotor symptoms.

Obstructive Sleep Apnea

Obstructive sleep apnea (OSA) is a common comorbidity of insomnia, with 55% to 84% of patients at sleep clinics presenting with symptoms of both conditions.[56] Insomnia is also associated with more severe OSA,[57] and initial and late insomnia often persist even after treatment for OSA.[58] Often, individuals with OSA are required to begin treatment with positive airway pressure (PAP) before beginning treatment for insomnia; however, this may result in increased frustration with the use of PAP machines and perhaps even decreased adherence.[56] A study of CBT-I and surgical interventions for mild OSA found that surgery improved symptoms of OSA more than CBT-I alone, but that CBT-I before surgery reduced sleep-onset difficulties.[59] A recent pilot study found that combining treatment for OSA with CBT-I led to significant clinical improvement in patients with both OSA and insomnia.[60] In at least one study, individuals with occult sleep-disordered breathing and insomnia experienced insomnia symptom relief similar to that of healthy controls after completing CBT-I.[61]

The presence of OSA alone should not rule out initiation of treatment with CBT-I,[62] and treatment for both conditions may be most effective when combined and when treated by a multidisciplinary team that can address patient questions.[56] Sleep restriction should be implemented cautiously in this population if there is significant daytime sleepiness.

Cancer

Insomnia is common among individuals with cancer diagnoses and those undergoing treatment for cancer. In breast cancer survivors, CBT-I has been demonstrated to be effective in treating insomnia,[63] and both in-person and telehealth delivery are effective in women with breast cancer.[64] Some patient characteristics may limit the efficacy of treatment, however, such as lower socioeconomic status and greater cancer severity.[65] The use of CBT-I versus pharmacologic interventions may be particularly helpful for patients who are already using multiple medications and may be at risk for drug interactions. Improvement in insomnia symptoms can greatly improve quality of life in cancer populations,[66] but further study in populations with specific cancer types is needed.

Emerging Areas

Cardiovascular disease and insomnia often co-occur. Indeed, almost 50% of individuals with chronic obstructive pulmonary disease also have sleep disturbances.[67] Studies suggest that insomnia likely contributes to the long-term risk of heart disease.[68] Although there are few studies examining the impact of CBT-I on patients with cardiovascular disease, one recent study found that CBT-I improved symptoms of insomnia and fatigue in individuals with stable heart failure; these effects were mediated by changes in beliefs and attitudes about sleep.[69] Herron and colleagues[70] also found improvement in insomnia symptoms and quality of life among a small sample of post-stroke patients with insomnia.

Traumatic brain injuries (TBI) are associated with a sequelae of symptoms that often include sleep disturbance, which could be a potential target for CBT-I. Because of disruptions to concentration and attention, some aspects of TBI might complicate the delivery of CBT-I. Unfortunately, there are few studies demonstrating the effectiveness of CBT-I in patients with TBI. Two case studies have had positive findings, however, indicating that CBT-I is a feasible intervention for some patients with TBI.[71,72] One randomized controlled trial found improved sleep among patients with TBI randomized to receive 8 sessions of CBT-I compared with a treatment as usual group.[73]

Conclusions

Growing evidence suggests that CBT-I can be a very effective adjunctive treatment to many medical conditions that co-occur with insomnia. Although evidence is limited that CBT-I might lead to improvement of medical conditions, findings indicate that reducing insomnia severity improves quality of life among individuals with comorbid medical conditions.[66,70] Treatment for insomnia may therefore be an important way to make progress toward delivering comprehensive care in these populations.

FUTURE DIRECTIONS

Insomnia is a cross-cutting disorder and precedes or accompanies numerous psychiatric and medical conditions. Recognition of how insomnia may increase risk for, or worsen, many conditions has increased in recent years and led to an emerging body of work focused on understanding the impact of treating insomnia when it co-occurs with other illnesses. The overarching results from randomized controlled trials summarized in a meta-analysis suggest that symptom improvement in comorbid psychiatric conditions seems to be more robust than in medical conditions after treatment with CBT-I.[7] This finding may be the result of common underlying causes between insomnia and psychiatric conditions, such as cognitive or emotional factors, that are specifically targeted by CBT-I.[7]

In order to understand more fully the role of comorbidity in treatment outcomes, future studies should use carefully considered inclusion criteria. For example, use of standardized assessment tools of insomnia (eg, Duke Structured Inventory for Sleep Disorders) and comorbid symptoms (eg, Structured Clinical Interview for DSM-5) would facilitate better characterization of the nature of these disorders, thereby allowing greater generalization of findings. Further, studies involving specific comorbid conditions should be replicated with larger samples because many have been underpowered to evaluate the comorbid symptoms. Importantly, these studies need to be large enough to evaluate adequately the comorbid condition as the primary outcome. More work is also needed to determine the mechanisms of action for the effects of CBT-I on both insomnia and symptoms of co-occurring conditions. In particular, better understanding of moderators of treatment success among the various comorbid conditions (eg, treatment responder vs failure patient characteristics) would allow the identification of those CBT-I components that are most likely to promote improvement. There is also a need for studies that more thoroughly address how insomnia affects comorbid conditions; for instance, determining whether improvements in comorbid symptoms are a direct effect of sleep improvement or if they are an indirect effect due to other aspects of the treatment.

Additional needs include research on multiple, concurrent comorbidities (eg, chronic pain AND depression) and how they might affect outcomes and treatment. Along these lines, future studies should specifically target sequencing CBT-I with treatments for various comorbid conditions to better inform stepwise or concurrent treatment. Indeed, CBT-I alone may be sufficient in some cases, and more efficient in treating some comorbid conditions than concurrent or stepwise treatment, but head-to-head randomized controlled trials are needed. There is a need for the integration of objective measures of sleep, particularly in the context of new research showing that those with both subjective and objective sleep impairments are the most severe insomnia subtype.[74]

Practical application of ongoing research requires the examination of efficacy of alternative delivery methods. Treatment for insomnia, with or without comorbidity, often requires highly specialized practitioners, which can create a bottleneck in service delivery or result in patients being treated late downstream in their illness. Further study is needed to inform treatment delivery through other providers such as primary care providers, nurses, and social workers.[38] There is also a need to develop more integrated treatments, where relevant sleep-focused interventions are combined with treatment for the comorbid condition. These might be informed by mechanistic studies understanding how insomnia affects other conditions.

The need for office visits may also affect patients' ability to receive care, as accessibility and transportation can prove significant obstacles, particularly for patients with comorbid conditions. Internet-based CBT-I has shown promise in improving both sleep and depression symptoms in populations with comorbid symptoms,[13,14] and telephone delivery had positive effects in perimenopausal women with insomnia.[55] It is important to understand comorbid symptoms before choosing the delivery system.[75] For instance, in patients with cancer, telemedicine may not be appropriate for treatment of those with severe symptoms.[64]

Based on a growing literature, CBT-I shows great promise in improving insomnia symptoms among populations with comorbid insomnia. Further, many studies have demonstrated marked improvements in nonsleep symptoms related to comorbid conditions after treatment with CBT-I. Continued thoughtful research should aim toward a better understanding of the mechanisms underlying improvement from CBT-I, with the eventual goal of using this intervention to treat co-occurring conditions as well as insomnia.

REFERENCES

1. Roth T, Coulouvrat C, Hajak G, et al. Prevalence and perceived health associated with insomnia based on DSM-IV-TR; International Statistical Classification of Diseases and Related Health Problems, Tenth Revision; and Research Diagnostic Criteria/International Classification of Sleep Disorders, Second Edition criteria: results from the America Insomnia Survey. Biol Psychiatry 2011;69(6):592–600.
2. Morin CM, LeBlanc M, Daley M, et al. Epidemiology of insomnia: prevalence, self-help treatments, consultations, and determinants of help-seeking behaviors. Sleep Med 2006;7(2):123–30.
3. Stewart R, Besset A, Bebbington P, et al. Insomnia comorbidity and impact and hypnotic use by age group in a national survey population aged 16 to 74 years. Sleep 2006;29(11):1391–7.
4. Ohayon MM, Roth T. Place of chronic insomnia in the course of depressive and anxiety disorders. J Psychiatr Res 2003;37(1):9–15.
5. Smith MT, Huang MI, Manber R. Cognitive behavior therapy for chronic insomnia occurring within the context of medical and psychiatric disorders. Clin Psychol Rev 2005;25(5):559–92.
6. Bei B, Ong JC, Rajaratnam SM, et al. Chronotype and improved sleep efficiency independently predict depressive symptom reduction after group cognitive behavioral therapy for insomnia. J Clin Sleep Med 2015;11(9):1021–7.
7. Wu JQ, Appleman ER, Salazar RD, et al. Cognitive behavioral therapy for insomnia comorbid with psychiatric and medical conditions: a meta-analysis. JAMA Intern Med 2015;175(9):1461–72.
8. Smith MT, Perlis ML. Who is a candidate for cognitive-behavioral therapy for insomnia? Health Psychol 2006;25(1):15–9.
9. McCurry SM, Logsdon RG, Teri L, et al. Evidence-based psychological treatments for insomnia in older adults. Psychol Aging 2007;22(1):18–27.
10. Manber R, Bernert RA, Suh S, et al. CBT for insomnia in patients with high and low depressive symptom severity: adherence and clinical outcomes. J Clin Sleep Med 2011;7(6):645–52.
11. Belanger L, Harvey AG, Fortier-Brochu E, et al. Impact of comorbid anxiety and depressive disorders on treatment response to cognitive behavior therapy for insomnia. J Consult Clin Psychol 2016;84(8):659–67.
12. van der Zweerde T, van Straten A, Effting M, et al. Does online insomnia treatment reduce depressive symptoms? A randomized controlled trial in individuals with both insomnia and depressive symptoms. Psychol Med 2019;49(3):501–9.
13. Batterham PJ, Christensen H, Mackinnon AJ, et al. Trajectories of change and long-term outcomes in a randomised controlled trial of internet-based insomnia treatment to prevent depression. BJPsych Open 2017;3(5):228–35.
14. Cheng P, Luik AI, Fellman-Couture C, et al. Efficacy of digital CBT for insomnia to reduce depression across demographic groups: a randomized trial. Psychol Med 2018;49(3):491–500.
15. Ong JC, Kuo TF, Manber R. Who is at risk for dropout from group cognitive-behavior therapy for insomnia? J Psychosom Res 2008;64(4):419–25.
16. Harvey AG, Schmidt DA, Scarna A, et al. Sleep-related functioning in euthymic patients with bipolar disorder, patients with insomnia, and subjects without sleep problems. Am J Psychiatry 2005;162(1):50–7.
17. Harvey AG, Soehner AM, Kaplan KA, et al. Treating insomnia improves mood state, sleep, and functioning in bipolar disorder: a pilot randomized controlled trial. J Consult Clin Psychol 2015;83(3):564–77.
18. Kaplan KA, Harvey AG. Behavioral treatment of insomnia in bipolar disorder. Am J Psychiatry 2013;170(7):716–20.
19. Lee KA. Alterations in sleep during pregnancy and postpartum: a review of 30 years of research. Sleep Med Rev 1998;2(4):231–42.
20. Okun ML, Roberts JM, Marsland AL, et al. How disturbed sleep may be a risk factor for adverse pregnancy outcomes. Obstet Gynecol Surv 2009;64(4):273–80.
21. Sedov ID, Goodman SH, Tomfohr-Madsen LM. Insomnia treatment preferences during pregnancy. J Obstet Gynecol Neonatal Nurs 2017;46(3):e95–104.
22. Tomfohr-Madsen LM, Clayborne ZM, Rouleau CR, et al. Sleeping for two: an open-pilot study of cognitive behavioral therapy for insomnia in pregnancy. Behav Sleep Med 2017;15(5):377–93.
23. Swanson LM, Flynn H, Adams-Mundy JD, et al. An open pilot of cognitive-behavioral therapy for insomnia in women with postpartum depression. Behav Sleep Med 2013;11(4):297–307.
24. Wallen GR, Brooks AT, Whiting B, et al. The prevalence of sleep disturbance in alcoholics admitted for treatment: a target for chronic disease management. Fam Community Health 2014;37(4):288–97.
25. Currie SR, Clark S, Hodgins DC, et al. Randomized controlled trial of brief cognitive-behavioural interventions for insomnia in recovering alcoholics. Addiction 2004;99(9):1121–32.
26. Arnedt JT, Conroy DA, Armitage R, et al. Cognitive-behavioral therapy for insomnia in alcohol dependent patients: a randomized controlled pilot trial. Behav Res Ther 2011;49(4):227–33.

27. Zhabenko O, Zhabenko NC, Conroy DA, et al. An open uncontrolled pilot trial of online cognitive-behavioral therapy for insomnia for Ukrainian alcohol-dependent patients. In: Andrade ALM, De Micheli D, editors. Innovations in the treatment of substance addiction. Cham (Switzerland): Springer International Publishing; 2016. p. 17.

28. Brower KJ. Assessment and treatment of insomnia in adult patients with alcohol use disorders. Alcohol 2015;49(4):417–27.

29. Schubert JR, Todd Arnedt J. Management of insomnia in patients with alcohol use disorder. Curr Sleep Med Rep 2017;3(2):38–47.

30. Currie SR, Clark S, Rimac S, et al. Comprehensive assessment of insomnia in recovering alcoholics using daily sleep diaries and ambulatory monitoring. Alcohol Clin Exp Res 2003;27(8): 1262–9.

31. Babson KA, Boden MT, Harris AH, et al. Poor sleep quality as a risk factor for lapse following a cannabis quit attempt. J Subst Abuse Treat 2013;44(4): 438–43.

32. Babson KA, Ramo DE, Baldini L, et al. Mobile app-delivered cognitive behavioral therapy for insomnia: feasibility and initial efficacy among veterans with cannabis use disorders. JMIR Res Protoc 2015; 4(3):e87.

33. Ohayon MM, Shapiro CM. Sleep disturbances and psychiatric disorders associated with posttraumatic stress disorder in the general population. Compr Psychiatry 2000;41(6):469–78.

34. Zayfert C, DeViva JC. Residual insomnia following cognitive behavioral therapy for PTSD. J Trauma Stress 2004;17(1):69–73.

35. Talbot LS, Maguen S, Metzler TJ, et al. Cognitive behavioral therapy for insomnia in posttraumatic stress disorder: a randomized controlled trial. Sleep 2014;37(2):327–41.

36. Kanady JC, Talbot LS, Maguen S, et al. Cognitive behavioral therapy for insomnia reduces fear of sleep in individuals with posttraumatic stress disorder. J Clin Sleep Med 2018;14(7):1193–203.

37. Vandrey R, Babson KA, Herrmann ES, et al. Interactions between disordered sleep, post-traumatic stress disorder, and substance use disorders. Int Rev Psychiatry 2014;26(2):237–47.

38. Manber R, Carney C, Edinger J, et al. Dissemination of CBTI to the non-sleep specialist: protocol development and training issues. J Clin Sleep Med 2012;8(2):209–18.

39. Ramsawh HJ, Stein MB, Belik SL, et al. Relationship of anxiety disorders, sleep quality, and functional impairment in a community sample. J Psychiatr Res 2009;43(10):926–33.

40. Belleville G, Ivers H, Belanger L, et al. Sequential treatment of comorbid insomnia and generalized anxiety disorder. J Clin Psychol 2016;72(9):880–96.

41. Taylor DJ, Pruiksma KE. Cognitive and behavioural therapy for insomnia (CBT-I) in psychiatric populations: a systematic review. Int Rev Psychiatry 2014; 26(2):205–13.

42. Edinger JD, Olsen MK, Stechuchak KM, et al. Cognitive behavioral therapy for patients with primary insomnia or insomnia associated predominantly with mixed psychiatric disorders: a randomized clinical trial. Sleep 2009;32(4):499–510.

43. Smith MT, Haythornthwaite JA. How do sleep disturbance and chronic pain inter-relate? Insights from the longitudinal and cognitive-behavioral clinical trials literature. Sleep Med Rev 2004;8(2):119–32.

44. Edinger JD, Wohlgemuth WK, Krystal AD, et al. Behavioral insomnia therapy for fibromyalgia patients: a randomized clinical trial. Arch Intern Med 2005;165(21):2527–35.

45. Currie SR, Wilson KG, Pontefract AJ, et al. Cognitive–behavioral treatment of insomnia secondary to chronic pain. J Consult Clin Psychol 2000;68(3): 407–16.

46. Finan PH, Buenaver LF, Coryell VT, et al. Cognitive-behavioral therapy for comorbid insomnia and chronic pain. Sleep Med Clin 2014;9(2):261–74.

47. Bohra MH, Espie CA. Is cognitive behavioural therapy for insomnia effective in treating insomnia and pain in individuals with chronic non-malignant pain? Br J Pain 2013;7(3):138–51.

48. Pigeon WR, Moynihan J, Matteson-Rusby S, et al. Comparative effectiveness of CBT interventions for co-morbid chronic pain & insomnia: a pilot study. Behav Res Ther 2012;50(11):685–9.

49. Xu Q, Lang CP. Examining the relationship between subjective sleep disturbance and menopause: a systematic review and meta-analysis. Menopause 2014;21(12):1301–18.

50. Baker FC, de Zambotti M, Colrain IM, et al. Sleep problems during the menopausal transition: prevalence, impact, and management challenges. Nat Sci Sleep 2018;10:73–95.

51. Arakane M, Castillo C, Rosero MF, et al. Factors relating to insomnia during the menopausal transition as evaluated by the Insomnia Severity Index. Maturitas 2011;69(2):157–61.

52. Galvan T, Camuso J, Sullivan K, et al. Association of estradiol with sleep apnea in depressed perimenopausal and postmenopausal women: a preliminary study. Menopause 2017;24(1):112–7.

53. Joffe H, Crawford SL, Freeman MP, et al. Independent contributions of nocturnal hot flashes and sleep disturbance to depression in estrogen-deprived women. J Clin Endocrinol Metab 2016;101(10): 3847–55.

54. Guthrie KA, Larson JC, Ensrud KE, et al. Effects of pharmacologic and nonpharmacologic interventions on insomnia symptoms and self-reported sleep quality in women with hot flashes: a pooled analysis

of individual participant data from four MsFLASH trials. Sleep 2018;41(1).

55. McCurry SM, Guthrie KA, Morin CM, et al. Telephone-based cognitive behavioral therapy for insomnia in perimenopausal and postmenopausal women with vasomotor symptoms: a MsFLASH randomized clinical trial. JAMA Intern Med 2016;176(7): 913–20.

56. Ong JC, Crawford MR, Kong A, et al. Management of obstructive sleep apnea and comorbid insomnia: a mixed-methods evaluation. Behav Sleep Med 2017;15(3):180–97.

57. Smith S, Sullivan K, Hopkins W, et al. Frequency of insomnia report in patients with obstructive sleep apnoea hypopnea syndrome (OSAHS). Sleep Med 2004;5(5):449–56.

58. Bjornsdottir E, Janson C, Sigurdsson JF, et al. Symptoms of insomnia among patients with obstructive sleep apnea before and after two years of positive airway pressure treatment. Sleep 2013;36(12): 1901–9.

59. Guilleminault C, Davis K, Huynh NT. Prospective randomized study of patients with insomnia and mild sleep disordered breathing. Sleep 2008;31(11): 1527–33.

60. Krakow B, Melendrez D, Lee SA, et al. Refractory insomnia and sleep-disordered breathing: a pilot study. Sleep Breath 2004;8(1):15–29.

61. Fung CH, Martin JL, Josephson K, et al. Efficacy of cognitive behavioral therapy for insomnia in older adults with occult sleep-disordered breathing. Psychosom Med 2016;78(5):629–39.

62. Sweetman A, Lack L, Lambert S, et al. Does comorbid obstructive sleep apnea impair the effectiveness of cognitive and behavioral therapy for insomnia? Sleep Med 2017;39:38–46.

63. Matthews EE, Berger AM, Schmiege SJ, et al. Cognitive behavioral therapy for insomnia outcomes in women after primary breast cancer treatment: a randomized, controlled trial. Oncol Nurs Forum 2014;41(3):241–53.

64. Savard J, Ivers H, Savard MH, et al. Long-term effects of two formats of cognitive behavioral therapy for insomnia comorbid with breast cancer. Sleep 2016;39(4):813–23.

65. Savard J, Savard MH, Ivers H. Moderators of treatment effects of a video-based cognitive-behavioral therapy for insomnia comorbid with cancer. Behav Sleep Med 2018;16(3):294–309.

66. Dirksen SR, Epstein DR. Efficacy of an insomnia intervention on fatigue, mood and quality of life in breast cancer survivors. J Adv Nurs 2008;61(6): 664–75.

67. Ohayon MM. Chronic Obstructive Pulmonary Disease and its association with sleep and mental disorders in the general population. J Psychiatr Res 2014;54:79–84.

68. Javaheri S, Redline S. Insomnia and risk of cardiovascular disease. Chest 2017;152(2):435–44.

69. Redeker NS, Jeon S, Andrews L, et al. Effects of cognitive behavioral therapy for insomnia on sleep-related cognitions among patients with stable heart failure. Behav Sleep Med 2017;1–13. [Epub ahead of print].

70. Herron K, Farquharson L, Wroe A, et al. Development and evaluation of a cognitive behavioural intervention for chronic post-stroke insomnia. Behav Cogn Psychother 2018;46(6):641–60.

71. Ouellet MC, Morin CM. Efficacy of cognitive-behavioral therapy for insomnia associated with traumatic brain injury: a single-case experimental design. Arch Phys Med Rehabil 2007;88(12): 1581–92.

72. Ouellet MC, Morin CM. Subjective and objective measures of insomnia in the context of traumatic brain injury: a preliminary study. Sleep Med 2006; 7(6):486–97.

73. Nguyen S, McKay A, Wong D, et al. Cognitive behavior therapy to treat sleep disturbance and fatigue after traumatic brain injury: a pilot randomized controlled trial. Arch Phys Med Rehabil 2017;98(8): 1508–17.e2.

74. Vgontzas AN, Fernandez-Mendoza J, Liao D, et al. Insomnia with objective short sleep duration: the most biologically severe phenotype of the disorder. Sleep Med Rev 2013;17(4):241–54.

75. Lancee J, Sorbi MJ, Eisma MC, et al. The effect of support on internet-delivered treatment for insomnia: does baseline depression severity matter? Behav Ther 2014;45(4):507–16.

Cognitive Behavioral Therapy for Insomnia in Depression

Lauren D. Asarnow, PhD[a],*, Rachel Manber, PhD[b]

KEYWORDS

- Depression • Insomnia • Comorbidity • Cognitive behavioral therapy for insomnia

KEY POINTS

- Recent research has expanded on previous research, which established that sleep problems are an important predictor of depression and that sleep problems are associated with more severe depression, more suicidality, and worse outcomes for treatment of depression.
- The relationship between sleep problems and depression is complex, likely bidirectional, and impactful.
- To further improve the lives of patients with depression who experience insomnia it will be important to investigate which patients will do better in a sequential versus concomitant approach.

The relationship between sleep and depression is bidirectional, complex, and apparent across the course of depression. Specifically, insomnia constitutes a risk for a future depressive episode among nondepressed individuals,[1] and its nocturnal symptoms are likely prodromal symptoms of depression among those who remitted from a depressive episode.[2] During depressive episodes as many as 67% to 84% of adults and 57% of children and adolescents report difficulties initiating or maintaining sleep,[3–5] and more severe insomnia symptoms are independently associated with greater functional impairment[6] and depressive symptom severity.[7] Persistence of insomnia symptoms is common among those with incomplete remission of depression (94.6%)[8] and even among those who fully remit following antidepressant therapy (72%)[9]; this suggests that treatment of depression does not provide sufficient sleep remedy. Furthermore, the presence of residual poor sleep among those who remit from depression constitutes a significant risk for a future depressive episode.[10,11]

The research reviewed in this article highlights some of the progress made over the past 5 years that elucidates this complex relationship between depression and insomnia as well as challenges in the treatment of insomnia when comorbid with depression. Overall, the data reviewed here support the idea that insomnia may be instigating, maintaining, and exacerbating depression.

POOR SLEEP PROSPECTIVELY PREDICTS DEPRESSION

Longitudinal epidemiologic studies in adults found that disturbed sleep and insomnia increase the risk of a future episode of major depressive disorder 1 to 3 years later (for reviews, see Franzen and Buysse[12] and Riemann and Voderholzer[13]). In a

Disclosure Statement: The authors certify that they have no affiliations with or financial involvement within the past 5 years and foreseeable future (eg, employment, consultancies, honoraria, stock ownership or options, expert testimony, grants or patents received or pending, royalties) with any organization or entity with a financial interest in or financial conflict with the subject matter or materials discussed in the article.
[a] Department of Psychiatry and Behavioral Sciences, Stanford University, 401 Quarry Road, Room 3342, Stanford, CA 94305, USA; [b] Department of Psychiatry and Behavioral Sciences, Stanford University, 401 Quarry Road, Room 3337, Stanford, CA 94305, USA
* Corresponding author.
E-mail address: lasarnow@stanford.edu

Sleep Med Clin 14 (2019) 177–184
https://doi.org/10.1016/j.jsmc.2019.01.009
1556-407X/19/© 2019 Elsevier Inc. All rights reserved.

2011 meta-analysis of 21 studies that prospectively evaluated poor sleep as a risk factor for a new depressive episode, Baglioni and colleagues[1] concluded that the presence of insomnia symptoms among adults without depression represents a significant risk for developing depression later. Four studies published since then are consistent with this conclusion. The first of these studies was a population-based sample of twins, which found that subjective poor sleep increased the risk of disability retirement for reasons of depression 10 to 20 years later.[14] The second was a large study of more than 24,000 adults, using prospective data collected at 2 time points 10 years apart.[15] The investigators found a bidirectional relationship between depression and insomnia symptoms.[15] The 3 other studies suggest that persistence of insomnia symptoms might be particularly relevant to the prediction of future depressive episodes. The first of these 2 studies was conducted among nondepressed adults in Korea and found that persistence of insomnia symptoms (in this study defined as insomnia at 2 or more time points) significantly increased the rate at which depression occurred over 6 years.[16] The second study, focused on a sample of community-dwelling older adults, found that persistent sleep disturbance (defined as presence of insomnia symptoms across 3 time points during a year-long period) was associated with depression the following year.[17] Lastly, a recent meta-analysis of 23 cross-sectional studies in older adults found that self-reported sleep disturbances increased the risk of the onset of depression (relative risk [RR] = 1.92) and persistent sleep disturbances increased the risk of the development (RR = 3.90), recurrence (RR = 7.70), and worsening (RR = 1.46) of depression in older adults.[18]

Research on poor sleep as a predictor of later depression in youth has lagged behind the adult literature but has increased in the past decade. Johnson and colleagues[19] found that, among youth aged 13 to 16 years with comorbid insomnia and depression, insomnia preceded depression in 69% of the sample; there was a significant association between prior insomnia and onset of depression even after adjusting for gender, race/ethnicity, and any prior anxiety disorder.[19] A study of 289 twin pairs found that sleep problems at age 8 predicted depression at age 10 years, with some indication that this association might be due to genes.[20] A recent review of the literature concluded that childhood sleep problems significantly predicted higher levels of depression, but not vice versa.[21] More recently, using data from the Great Smoky Mountains Study, the investigators found a bidirectional relationship between sleep and depression, such that sleep problems

during childhood predicted increases in the prevalence of later depression and anxiety symptoms in adolescents, and depression in childhood predicted increases in sleep problems over time.[22] We examined specific sleep parameters that predict future depressive episodes using a nationally representative sample of adolescents. We found that late bedtime in middle school predicted more depression symptoms in young adulthood.[23]

Poor Sleep Prospectively Predicts Suicidality and Self-Harm

Results from a recent meta-analysis indicate that, among adults, insomnia is also a prospective risk factor for suicidal ideation, suicidal behavior, and completed suicide, even in studies that adjusted for the presence or absence of depressive disorder or symptoms.[24] A later study similarly found that persistent insomnia (defined as the presence of insomnia at 2 or more time points) among individuals without a depression diagnosis at baseline increases the risk of suicidal thoughts across the span of 6 years.[16] The research regarding the relationship between sleep and suicidality and self-harm in adolescents is consistent with the adult literature. Self-reported difficulties initiating or maintaining sleep at ages 12 to 14 years significantly predicted suicidal thoughts and self-harm behaviors at ages 15 to 17 years.[25]

POOR SLEEP ASSOCIATED WITH MORE SEVERE DEPRESSION, INCLUDING SUICIDALITY

Depressive symptom severity is positively associated with insomnia symptom severity. For example, in the National Comorbidity Study—Revision data, the presence of insomnia symptoms (difficulty initiating or maintaining sleep determined using the Quick Inventory of Depressive Symptoms—Self Report)[26] was associated with more severe symptoms of depression.[6] Severity of depressive symptoms is also positively associated with objective indices of sleep disturbance. For example, among postpartum women, objective (actigraphic) measures of difficulties maintaining sleep (eg, sleep fragmentation, sleep efficiency, and time awake after sleep onset) were significantly correlated with severity of depressive symptoms.[27] The association between severity of depressive symptoms and poor sleep has also been documented among youth.[5]

Poor sleep is also associated with elevation in specific symptoms of depression. For example, Emslie and colleagues[5] found that among children and adolescents with depressive disorders, insomnia symptoms, which were present in more than half of the sample, were associated with greater severity of specific depressive symptoms, including fatigue, suicidal ideation, physical complaints, and concentration. Similarly among college students with depressive symptoms, those reporting sleep disturbance had more anxiety symptoms than those without sleep disturbance.[28]

Poor Sleep Associated with Suicidality in Adults and Youth

Controlling for depressive symptoms, poor subjective sleep quality at baseline was associated with increased risk for death by suicide at a 10-year follow-up in a population-based community sample of older adults.[29] Two recent publications also examined the relationship between objective sleep measures derived from sleep laboratory polysomnography and suicidal ideation among adults with treatment-resistant depression. The first study found that greater nocturnal wakefulness, particularly in the early-morning hours (eg, during the 4:00 AM hour), was significantly associated with next-day suicidal thoughts adjusting for depression severity.[30] Secondary analysis of the same data found that, independent of depression severity, suicidal ideation was associated with specific sleep architecture; specifically less non–rapid eye movement (REM) stage 4 sleep and more time awake in the middle of the night across groups with bipolar and unipolar depression.[31]

In children and adolescents, recent research has extended past research[32] documenting the connection between sleep and suicidal ideation and self-harm by examining several specific subjective sleep complaints (ie, difficulty maintaining sleep, sleep difficulty bedtime variability, short sleep duration, and nonrestorative sleep). One study of more than 600 school-aged children from the community found that significantly more children with self-harm behaviors reported subjective difficulty maintaining sleep after adjusting for symptoms of depression.[33] A cross-sectional, national, and representative sample consisting of more than 75,000 students (grades 7 to 12) in Korea found that nonrestorative sleep and short sleep duration were significantly associated with suicidal ideation in adolescents.[34] In another study, using a distinct sample of Korean adolescents, weekend catch-up sleep duration (an indicator of insufficient weekday sleep) was associated with suicide attempts and self-injury.[35]

POOR SLEEP ASSOCIATED WITH POOR RESPONSE TO DEPRESSION TREATMENTS

The body of research on the relationship between treatment response to both psychotherapy and psychopharmacologic treatment of depression and subjective and objective measures of sleep is growing. Subjective and objectively measured sleep disturbance predict attrition and remission rates as well as stability of psychopharmacologic depression treatment response.[36–38] The literature also documents persistent insomnia symptoms as a risk factor for recurrence of depression symptoms following treatment with interpersonal psychotherapy, despite continued maintenance treatment.[10] Another study reports that patients with objectively measured sleep abnormalities (early REM latency, low sleep efficiency, and greater REM density) who were treated with interpersonal psychotherapy had worse remission rates than those with more typical sleep profiles.[39] More recently, a pooled sample of more than 700 adult outpatients with depression drawn from 6 clinical trials at the University of Pittsburgh between 1982 and 2001 examined the association between objectively measured sleep parameters (via polysomnography) and remission from pharmacologic (imipramine, nortriptyline, fluoxetine, paroxetine, or bupropion) and/or psychological (interpersonal therapy or cognitive behavioral therapy) treatments of depression.[40] The study found that prolonged sleep latency (>30 minutes) and shorter sleep duration ($\leq$6 hours) alone or in combination with insomnia predicted an increased risk of nonremission (remission defined as a Hamilton Depression Rating Scale score of $\leq$7) and that patients with 3 or more baseline sleep disturbances were 3 times less likely to reach remission.[40]

It is interesting that recent research in children and adolescents points to differences in antidepressant treatment response in those with and without insomnia symptoms by age group. One study in 166 depressed adolescents treated with a 12-week course of sertraline, cognitive behavioral therapy, or their combination found that across treatment groups, lower response and remission rates were associated with pretreatment and ongoing sleep disturbance across treatment groups.[41] Another study of both children and adolescents treated with fluoxetine found that although response rates were similar in those with or without insomnia symptoms, there was a significant difference by age group; among adolescents, those with insomnia symptoms were less likely to respond to fluoxetine than those without, whereas in children the reverse was true: those with insomnia symptoms were more likely to respond to fluoxetine than those without insomnia.[5] It is not clear why age moderated the association between disturbed sleep and baseline and response to fluoxetine. The investigators suggest that this might be related to developmental differences in sleep architecture between depressed children and adolescents.[5]

Therapeutic Strategies

There are effective pharmacologic and nonpharmacologic treatments for both insomnia and depression. The treatment of comorbid depression and insomnia involves clinical decisions about which and in what order to introduce the treatments for the 2 disorders. Here we focus our discussion on evidence concerning the order of treatments for the 2 disorders, leaving out the complex issues involved in selection of specific medications and specific psychotherapies. We note that research on the question of sequencing included mainly cognitive behavioral therapy for insomnia (CBT-I) and for depression (CBT-D), and interpersonal therapy for depression (IPT).

SEQUENTIAL TREATMENT

One strategy for treating patients with insomnia-depression comorbidity is to treat one disorder at a time. As reviewed earlier, starting the sequence with depression treatment alone will likely leave many with unresolved insomnia symptoms. As residual insomnia symptoms constitute a risk for relapse and recurrence, it important to treat them.[42] Watanabe and colleagues[43] provide preliminary promising results in a pilot study that evaluated the strategy of adding a brief (4 sessions) behavioral therapy for insomnia to usual care of patients who did not fully remit with pharmacotherapy for depression and experienced residual insomnia symptoms. The study found significant improvement in insomnia and depression symptoms, with large effect sizes relative to treatment as usual (number needed to treat = 2). In another pilot study, Ashworth and colleagues[44] compared 4 sessions of face-to-face CBT-I with self-help CBT-I for patients experiencing residual insomnia symptoms after being treated with antidepressants for at least 6 weeks. The results indicate that those treated with face-to-face CBT-I experienced greater improvement in insomnia and depression severity.[44] It will be important to follow these promising results with larger studies and longer follow-up that can evaluate whether these sequential strategies positively affect the course of depression over time by reducing the risk or shortening the time to relapse and recurrence.

Because research on the strategy of first treating insomnia is hindered by ethical challenges, studies evaluating the efficacy of this strategy included only patients with milder depression and were short term.[11,45] One exception is a recent small study that compared how patients with a dual diagnosis of insomnia and major depressive disorder responded to 9 weeks of online treatments with either CBT-I (n = 22) or CBT-D (n = 21).[46] Results indicated that online CBT-I was significantly more effective than treatment of depression in improving insomnia (57% versus 19% of treatment completers no longer met criteria for insomnia) and comparable in reducing depression (37% versus 21% of completers no longer met depression criteria).[46] These preliminary results cannot be interpreted because of the small sample and importantly also because there is a differential rate of completion of the 2 online treatments. One controlled and several uncontrolled studies of group CBT-I also found significant improvements in both insomnia and depression after treatment. Norell-Clarke and colleagues[47] investigated the effects of group CBT-I on insomnia and depressive symptomatology in a comorbid sample through a randomized controlled trial. The investigators found that CBT-I was more efficient than a control treatment in reducing insomnia severity and that CBT-I was associated with a higher proportion of remission from both insomnia and depression diagnoses than a control treatment. Ong and colleagues[48] reported that group CBT-I among patients seeking treatment for insomnia in a sleep center was equally effective for those with and without elevation in depressive symptom severity, and led to modest reduction in depression severity and suicidal ideation.

CONCOMITANT TREATMENT

Another strategy for the treatment of depression-insomnia comorbidity is to treat both disorders concomitantly. This strategy has the advantage of more rapid reduction of suffering because patients could achieve relief of depression insomnia earlier than they would with the sequential approach. Here we review results from studies that evaluated the concomitant treatment strategy, examining the effects of this strategy on both disorders. Randomized controlled studies clearly indicate that combining antidepressant medications with CBT-I effectively alleviates insomnia symptoms in adults[49,50] and adolescents.[51] Results pertaining to the effects of the concomitant approach on depression outcomes have been mixed. In an earlier randomized controlled pilot study, the authors found that combining escitalopram with CBT-I improved remission from depression relative to escitalopram plus active control therapy for insomnia among adults with comorbid insomnia and major depressive disorder.[49] However, the subsequent larger randomized controlled trial, the Treatment of Insomnia in Depression (TRIAD), did not replicate the results from the pilot study. The TRIAD study randomized individuals to receive an antidepressant pharmacotherapy algorithm with either CBT-I or the same control therapy as in the pilot study, and found no difference in depression remission.[50] However, further analysis revealed that improvements in insomnia at week 6 of treatment mediated eventual remission from depression.[50] Similarly, in a randomized controlled trial that compared escitalopram plus CBT-I with either CBT-I plus placebo tablet or escitalopram plus 4-session sleep hygiene control in adults with major depressive disorder and insomnia disorder, Carney and colleagues[52] found that although all groups' self-reported sleep improved, only the CBT-I groups improved on objective sleep, and sleep worsened in the group that received antidepressants plus sleep hygiene. Although depression symptoms across all groups improved significantly from baseline to post-treatment, the change in depression symptoms from baseline to post-treatment did not differ between groups.

Similar to negative findings in adults, a pilot randomized controlled trial in adolescents also failed to show benefits of adding CBT-I to treatment of depression. The study compared the combination of CBT-D plus CBT-I with CBT-D plus sleep hygiene control therapy for insomnia among adolescents with comorbid insomnia and depression, and found no difference in rates of recovery from depression between the 2 conditions.[51] However, when limiting the analysis to those who remitted from depression, the researchers found a trend for faster remission among those in the CBT-I condition.[51]

The concomitant strategy also has the potential to affect patients' tolerance of antidepressant medications. The TRIAD study reported that CBT-I participants reported greater frequency of medication side effects and higher maximum side effect than participants randomized to the control insomnia therapy. However, no participant discontinued the study because of antidepressant side effects.[50]

CHALLENGES TREATING INSOMNIA COMORBID WITH DEPRESSION

Although, as reviewed in the previous section, CBT-I is efficacious for the treatment of insomnia comorbid with depression, treating insomnia comorbid with depression presents some unique challenges. Indeed, among patients participating in group CBT-I in a sleep clinic, those with elevated depressive symptom severity are more likely to

discontinue treatment.[48] Moreover, a study from Edinger and colleagues[53] found that patients with comorbid depression and insomnia who experienced the first onset of both disorders in childhood are less responsive to CBT-I than are those with their first onset as an adult. Also, the literature suggests that individuals with insomnia comorbid with depression may be at increased risk for poor adherence and response. We review here some of these risks and suggest strategies for addressing the challenges that they present when implementing CBT-I.

Cognitions

Research indicates that patients with insomnia and depression report more unhelpful beliefs about sleep than those who experience insomnia without comorbid depression,[54] and that such beliefs are linked to more treatment-resistant insomnia.[55–57] Maladaptive beliefs about sleep might also serve as barriers to engagement and adherence to some treatment recommendations.[58] For example, a belief that 8 hours of sleep is required in order to function can lead to increased anxiety and low engagement and/or adherence when the recommended time in bed is restricted to less than the desired amount. Rumination, which is common in depression,[59] is associated with worse sleep quality[60] and a tendency to ruminate about daytime consequences of insomnia.[60] Maladaptive beliefs and rumination that are common in depression can be addressed using cognitive therapy.

Anhedonia

Some persons with depression find it difficult to make the behavioral changes necessary for improving their sleep. These individuals go to bed earlier than when euthymic, get out of bed later, or both because they do not enjoy activities that were previously pleasurable or rewarding and/or as an escape from emotional suffering.[61] This makes it difficult to adhere to core treatment recommendations, such as sleep restriction[62] and stimulus control instructions.[63] Behavioral activation[64] can be used to overcome these barriers to adherence. Behavioral activation involves helping depressed people re-engage in their lives through focused activation strategies that counter patterns of avoidance, withdrawal, and inactivity that may exacerbate depressive episodes, replacing them with opportunities to help individuals approach and access sources of positive reinforcement in their lives, which can serve a natural antidepressant function; it is an integral component of CBT-D. In the context of insomnia, behavioral activation is focused primarily on pre-bedtime behavior to facilitate postponing bedtime, and in the morning to facilitate getting out of bed at the recommended time.

SUMMARY

In conclusion, the relationship between sleep problems and depression is complex, likely bidirectional, and impactful. The adult and adolescent literature points to the presence of insomnia symptoms as an important predictor and/or precursor to a depressive episode. Moreover, insomnia symptoms are associated with more severe symptoms of depression, including increased suicidality, and predict poor treatment response in depressive adults and adolescents. Fortunately, CBT-I is an effective short-term treatment of insomnia symptoms when depression and insomnia symptoms are co-occurring. In the past 5 years research has taken 2 approaches to treating comorbid insomnia and depression symptoms: a sequential approach, whereby providers treat one disorder at a time, or a concomitant approach whereby both disorders are treated simultaneously. Although initial results from studies that assessed the sequential approach (treating either insomnia before depression treatment or treating residual insomnia symptoms following depression treatment) have been promising, more adequately powered randomized controlled trials with long-term follow-up are needed to evaluate how sequential strategies affect the course of depression over time. The literature on whether concomitant treatment of depression and insomnia results in improved depression outcomes is also in its nascent stages, with mixed results. Nonetheless, a recent finding that response to insomnia treatment mediated eventual remission from depression suggests that a focused effort to improve insomnia has the potential to enhance the outcomes of depression treatment. To further improve the lives of patients with depression who experience insomnia, it will be important to investigate which patients will do better in a sequential versus concomitant approach.

REFERENCES

1. Baglioni C, Battagliese G, Feige B, et al. Insomnia as a predictor of depression: a meta-analytic evaluation of longitudinal epidemiological studies. J Affect Disord 2011;135(1-3):10–9.
2. Perlis ML, Giles DE, Buysse DJ, Tu X, Kupfer DJ. Self-reported sleep disturbance as a prodromal symptom in recurrent depression. J Affect Disord 1997;42(2-3):209–12.
3. Hamilton M. Frequency of symptoms in melancholia (depressive illness). Br J Psychiatry 1989;154:201–6.
4. Ford DE, Kamerow DB. Epidemiologic study of sleep disturbances and psychiatric disorders. An opportunity for prevention? JAMA 1989;262(11):1479–84.
5. Emslie GJ, Kennard BD, Mayes TL, et al. Insomnia moderates outcome of serotonin-selective reuptake inhibitor treatment in depressed youth. J Child and Adolesc Psychopharmacol 2012;22(1):21–8.
6. Soehner AM, Kaplan KA, Harvey AG. Prevalence and clinical correlates of co-occurring insomnia and hypersomnia symptoms in depression. J Affect Disord 2014;167:93–7.
7. Taylor DJ, Lichstein KL, Durrence HH, Reidel BW, Bush AJ. Epidemiology of insomnia, depression, and anxiety. Sleep 2005;28(11):1457–64.
8. McClintock SM, Husain MM, Wisniewski SR, et al. Residual symptoms in depressed outpatients who respond by 50% but do not remit to antidepressant medication. J Clin Psychopharmacol 2011;31(2):180–6.
9. Nierenberg AA, Husain MM, Trivedi MH, et al. Residual symptoms after remission of major depressive disorder with citalopram and risk of relapse: a STAR*D report. Psychological Medicine 2010;40(1):41–50.
10. Dombrovski AY, Cyranowski JM, Mulsant BH, et al. Which symptoms predict recurrence of depression in women treated with maintenance interpersonal psychotherapy? Depress Anxiety 2008;25(12):1060–6.
11. Taylor DJ, Walters HM, Vittengl JR, et al. Which depressive symptoms remain after response to cognitive therapy of depression and predict relapse and recurrence? J Affect Disord 2010;123(1–3):181–7.
12. Franzen PL, Buysse DJ. Sleep disturbances and depression: risk relationships for subsequent depression and therapeutic implications. Dialogues Clin Neurosci 2008;10(4):473–81.
13. Riemann D, Voderholzer U. Primary insomnia: a risk factor to develop depression? J Affect Disord 2003;76(1–3):255–9.
14. Paunio T, Korhonen T, Hublin C, et al. Poor sleep predicts symptoms of depression and disability retirement due to depression. J Affect Disord 2015;172:381–9.
15. Sivertsen B, Salo P, Mykletun A, et al. The bidirectional association between depression and insomnia: the HUNT study. Psychosom Med 2012;74(7):758–65.
16. Suh S, Kim H, Yang H-C, et al. Longitudinal course of depression scores with and without insomnia in non-depressed individuals: a 6-year follow-up longitudinal study in a Korean cohort. Sleep 2013;36(3):369–76.

17. Lee E, Cho HJ, Olmstead R, et al. Persistent sleep disturbance: a risk factor for recurrent depression in community-dwelling older adults. Sleep 2013; 36(11):1685–91.

18. Bao YP, Han Y, Ma J, et al. Cooccurrence and bidirectional prediction of sleep disturbances and depression in older adults: meta-analysis and systematic review. Neurosci Biobehav Rev 2017;75: 257–73.

19. Johnson EO, Roth T, Breslau N. The association of insomnia with anxiety disorders and depression: exploration of the direction of risk. J Psychiatr Res 2006;40(8):700–8.

20. Gregory AM, Rijsdijk FV, Lau JYF, et al. The direction of longitudinal associations between sleep problems and depression symptoms: a study of twins aged 8 and 10 years. Sleep 2009;32(2):189–99.

21. Alvaro PK, Roberts RM, Harris JK. A systematic review assessing bidirectionality between sleep disturbances, anxiety, and depression. Sleep 2013;36(7): 1059–68.

22. Shanahan L, Copeland WE, Angold A, et al. Sleep problems predict and are predicted by generalized anxiety/depression and oppositional defiant disorder. J Am Acad Child Adolesc Psychiatry 2014; 53(5):550–8.

23. Asarnow LD, McGlinchey E, Harvey AG. The effects of bedtime and sleep duration on academic and emotional outcomes in a nationally representative sample of adolescents. J Adolesc Health 2014; 54(3):350–6.

24. Pigeon WR, Pinquart M, Conner K. Meta-analysis of sleep disturbance and suicidal thoughts and behaviors. J Clin Psychiatry 2012;73(9):e1160–7.

25. Wong MM, Brower KJ, Zucker RA. Sleep problems, suicidal ideation, and self-harm behaviors in adolescence. J Psychiatr Res 2011;45(4):505–11.

26. Manber R, Blasey C, Arnow B, et al. Assessing insomnia severity in depression: comparison of depression rating scales and sleep diaries. J Psychiatr Res 2005;39(5):481–8.

27. Park EM, Meltzer-Brody S, Stickgold R. Poor sleep maintenance and subjective sleep quality are associated with postpartum maternal depression symptom severity. Arch Womens Ment Health 2013; 16(6):539–47.

28. Nyer M, Farabaugh A, Fehling K, et al. Relationship between sleep disturbance and depression, anxiety, and functioning in college students. Depress Anxiety 2013;30(9):873–80.

29. Bernert RA, Turvey CL, Conwell Y, et al. Association of poor subjective sleep quality with risk for death by suicide during a 10-year period a longitudinal, population-based study of late life. JAMA Psychiatry 2014;71(10):1129–37.

30. Ballard ED, Vande Voort JL, Bernert RA, et al. Nocturnal wakefulness is associated with next-day suicidal ideation in major depressive disorder and bipolar disorder. J Clin Psychiatry 2016;77(6): 825–31.

31. Bernert RA, Luckenbaugh DA, Duncan WC, et al. Sleep architecture parameters as a putative biomarker of suicidal ideation in treatment-resistant depression. J Affect Disord 2017;208:309–15.

32. Goldstein TR, Bridge JA, Brent DA. Sleep disturbance preceding completed suicide in adolescents. J Consult Clin Psychol 2008;76(1):84–91.

33. Singareddy R, Krishnamurthy VB, Vgontzas AN, et al. Subjective and objective sleep and self-harm behaviors in young children: a general population study. Psychiatry Res 2013;209(3):549–53.

34. Park JH, Yoo JH, Kim SH. Associations between non-restorative sleep, short sleep duration and suicidality: findings from a representative sample of Korean adolescents. Psychiatry Clin Neurosci 2013;67(1):28–34.

35. Kang SG, Lee YJ, Kim SJ, et al. Weekend catch-up sleep is independently associated with suicide attempts and self-injury in Korean adolescents. Compr Psychiatry 2014;55(2):319–25.

36. Buysse DJ, Reynolds CF, Houck PR, et al. Does lorazepam impair the antidepressant response to nortriptyline and psychotherapy? J Clin Psychiatry 1997;58(10):426–32.

37. Dew MA, Reynolds CF, Houck PR, et al. Temporal profiles of the course of depression during treatment: predictors of pathways toward recovery in the elderly. Arch Gen Psychiatry 1997;54(11): 1016–24.

38. Thase ME. Depression, sleep, and antidepressants. J Clin Psychiatry 1998;59(Suppl 4):55–65.

39. Thase ME, Fasiczka AL, Berman SR, et al. Electroencephalographic sleep profiles before and after cognitive behavior therapy of depression. Arch Gen Psychiatry 1998;55(2):138–44.

40. Troxel WM, Kupfer DJ, Reynolds CF, et al. Insomnia and objectively measured sleep disturbances predict treatment outcome in depressed patients treated with psychotherapy or psychotherapy- pharmacotherapy combinations. J Clin Psychiatry 2012; 73(4):478–85.

41. Manglick M, Rajaratnam SM, Taffe J, et al. Persistent sleep disturbance is associated with treatment response in adolescents with depression. Aust N Z J Psychiatry 2013;47(6):556–63.

42. Kurian BT, Greer TL, Trivedi MH. Strategies to enhance the therapeutic efficacy of antidepressants: targeting residual symptoms. Expert Rev Neurother 2009;9(7):975–84.

43. Watanabe N, Furukawa TA, Shimodera S, et al. Brief behavioral therapy for refractory insomnia in residual depression: an assessor-blind, randomized controlled trial. J Clin Psychiatry 2011; 72(12):1651–8.

44. Ashworth DK, Sletten TL, Junge M, et al. A randomized controlled trial of cognitive behavioral therapy for insomnia: an effective treatment for comorbid insomnia and depression. J Couns Psychol 2015;62(2):115–23.

45. Manber R, Bernert RA, Suh S, et al. CBT for insomnia in patients with high and low depressive symptom severity: adherence and clinical outcomes. J Clin Sleep Med 2011;7(6):645–52.

46. Blom K, Jernelöv S, Kraepelien M, et al. Internet treatment addressing either insomnia or depression, for patients with both diagnoses: a randomized trial. Sleep 2015;38(2):267–77.

47. Norell-Clarke A, Jansson-Fröjmark M, Tillfors M, et al. Group cognitive behavioural therapy for insomnia: effects on sleep and depressive symptomatology in a sample with comorbidity. Behav Res Ther 2015;74:80–93.

48. Ong JC, Kuo TF, Manber R. Who is at risk for dropout from group cognitive-behavior therapy for insomnia? J Psychosom Res 2008;64(4):419–25.

49. Manber R, Edinger JD, Gress JL, et al. Cognitive behavioral therapy for insomnia enhances depression outcome in patients with comorbid major depressive disorder and insomnia. Sleep 2008; 31(4):489–95.

50. Manber R, Buysse DJ, Edinger J, et al. Efficacy of cognitive-behavioral therapy for insomnia combined with antidepressant pharmacotherapy in patients with comorbid depression and insomnia: a randomized controlled trial. J Clin Psychiatry 2016;77(10): e1316–23.

51. Clarke G, McGlinchey EL, Hein K, et al. Cognitive-behavioral treatment of insomnia and depression in adolescents: a pilot randomized trial. Behav Res Ther 2015;69:111–8.

52. Carney CE, Edinger JD, Kuchibhatla M, et al. Cognitive behavioral insomnia therapy for those with insomnia and depression: a randomized controlled clinical trial. Sleep 2017;40(4). https://doi.org/10.1093/sleep/zsx019.

53. Edinger JD, Manber R, Buysse DJ, et al. Are patients with childhood onset of insomnia and depression more difficult to treat than are those with adult onsets of these disorders? A report from the TRIAD study. J Clin Sleep Med 2017;13(2):205–13.

54. Carney CE, Edinger JD, Manber R, et al. Beliefs about sleep in disorders characterized by sleep and mood disturbance. J Psychosom Res 2007; 62(2):179–88.

55. Morin CM, Blais F, Savard J. Are changes in beliefs and attitudes about sleep related to sleep improvements in the treatment of insomnia? Behav Res Ther 2002;40(7):741–52.

56. Tremblay V, Savard J, Ivers H. Predictors of the effect of cognitive behavioral therapy for chronic insomnia comorbid with breast cancer. J Consult Clin Psychol 2009;77(4):742–50.

57. Cvengros JA, Crawford MR, Manber R, et al. The relationship between beliefs about sleep and adherence to behavioral treatment combined with meditation for insomnia. Behav Sleep Med 2015;13(1): 52–63.

58. Carney CE, Edinger JD. Identifying critical beliefs about sleep in primary insomnia. Sleep 2006;29(4): 444–53.

59. Thomsen DK, Mehlsen MY, Christensen S, et al. Rumination—relationship with negative mood and sleep quality. Pers Indiv Differ 2003;34(7):1293–301.

60. Carney CE, Edinger JD, Meyer B, et al. Symptom-focused rumination and sleep disturbance. Behav Sleep Med 2006;4(4):228–41.

61. Hauri P, Fisher J. Persistent psychophysiologic (learned) insomnia. Sleep 1986;9(1):38–53.

62. Spielman AJJ, Saskin P, Thorpy MJJ. Treatment of chronic insomnia by restriction of time in bed. Sleep 1987;10(1):45–56.

63. Bootzin RR, Epstein D, Wood JM. Stimulus control instructions. In: Hauri P, editor. Case studies in insomnia. New York: Springer; 1991. p. 19–28.

64. Jacobson NS, Martell CR, Dimidjian S. Behavioral activation treatment for depression: returning to contextual roots. Clin Psychol Sci Pract 2006;8(3): 255–70.

Cognitive Behavioral Therapy for Insomnia and Women's Health
Sex as a Biological Variable

Sara Nowakowski, PhD[a],*, Jessica M. Meers, MA[b]

KEYWORDS

- Sleep • Insomnia • Women • Pregnancy • Postpartum • Menopause

KEY POINTS

- Differences in sleep for men and women begin at a very early age, with women reporting poorer sleep and having a higher risk for insomnia compared with men.
- Women are particularly vulnerable to developing insomnia during times of reproductive hormonal change.
- Sleep across the woman's lifespan and special treatment considerations for using cognitive behavioral therapy for insomnia (CBT-I) in women will be addressed in this review.

INTRODUCTION

Several studies have demonstrated that women report more sleep difficulties[1,2] and are at greater risk for a diagnosis of insomnia compared with men.[3,4] In the National Sleep Foundation's 2007 poll, 30% of pregnant women and 42% of postpartum women reported rarely getting a good night's sleep, compared with 15% among all women. In addition, 25% of perimenopausal women and 30% of postmenopausal women reported getting a good night's sleep only a few nights per month or less.[5,6] In general, there is a higher prevalence of insomnia and dissatisfaction with sleep in women. In contrast, objective measures of sleep, measured by actigraphy and polysomnography (PSG), have demonstrated shorter sleep onset latency, increased sleep efficiency, and total sleep time in women compared with men.[7–9] A meta-analysis of sex differences of sleep behaviors in older adults (aged 58+) revealed no sex differences in total sleep time.[10] Although sleep disturbances and insomnia disorder are widespread in the general population, they tend to occur more frequently in women, particularly during times of hormonal fluctuation. In addition to sex differences found in the complaint of sleep disturbances and prevalence of insomnia, sex differences also exist for the treatment of sleep complaints. For example, in 2013 the US Food and Drug Administration required the manufacturers of Ambien to lower the recommended dose of zolpidem for women from 10 to 5 mg for immediate-release products, and from 12.5 to 6.25 mg for extended-release products, because of the risk of next-morning impairment and motor vehicle accidents. Women seem to be more susceptible to this risk because they eliminate zolpidem from their bodies more slowly than men. Zolpidem is the first drug in the United States to have different recommended doses for women versus men, but it seems likely that pharmacokinetic sex differences would lead to differences in rates of absorption, metabolism, and excretion of other medications

Conflicts of Interest: None.

[a] Department of Obstetrics and Gynecology, University of Texas Medical Branch, 301 University Boulevard, Galveston, TX 77555-0587, USA; [b] Department of Psychology, University of Houston, 4800 Calhoun Road, Houston, TX 77204, USA

* Corresponding author.

E-mail address: sanowako@utmb.edu

as well. Other biopsychosocial factors, such as discomfort during pregnancy, breastfeeding, and infant/child care during the postpartum period, and potential ongoing nocturnal vasomotor symptoms (hot flashes and night sweats) during peri- and postmenopause, may complicate insomnia treatment and require special treatment considerations for sleep disturbances in women.

THE MENSTRUAL CYCLE AND MENSTRUAL CYCLE DISORDERS

The menstrual cycle of healthy women is characterized by cyclic changes in production of estradiol, progesterone, lutenizing hormone, follicle-stimulating hormone, prolactin, and growth hormone. Reproductive hormones not only regulate reproductive function during the menstrual cycle, but also influence sleep and circadian rhythms. Negative menstrual symptoms are most commonly experienced by women during the last few days of the cycle, as progesterone and estrogen levels decline.[11] **(Fig. 1)**.

Premenstrual syndrome (PMS) and premenstrual dysphoric disorder (PMDD) are characterized by emotional, behavioral, and physical symptoms that occur in the premenstrual phase of the menstrual cycle, with resolution at the onset of menses or shortly thereafter. Many women of reproductive age experience some premenstrual symptoms, but 3% to 8% of women have clinically relevant premenstrual symptoms that they perceive as distressing and that affect daily function and meet diagnostic criteria.[6,12–14] Women with PMS/PMDD typically report sleep-related complaints such as insomnia, frequent awakenings, non-restorative sleep, unpleasant dreams or nightmares, and poor sleep quality associated with their symptoms; and daytime disturbances such as sleepiness,

fatigue, decreased alertness, and an inability to concentrate during the during the premenstrual week and during the first few days of menstruation.[15–24] Women who experience severe PMS report significant declines in sleep quality in association with their symptoms during the late luteal phase compared with the early follicular phase of their cycle.[25–27] Changes in progesterone and estrogen, rather than absolute levels, in the late luteal phase may be an important consideration in determining factors associated with sleep quality. Actigraphic sleep was examined in participants from the Study of Women's Health Across the Nationand investigators found that, among later-reproductive-age women, sleep efficiency and total sleep time declines across the menstrual cycle, with the most pronounced decline in the last week of the menstrual cycle.[28] These corresponding changes, however, were not found in PSG sleep.[29–31] Another study demonstrated that a steeper rate of increase in progesterone levels from follicular phase through mid luteal phase was associated with greater PSG wake after sleep onset and sleep fragmentation in the late luteal phase.[32] Sleep studies across the menstrual cycle have been limited by small sample sizes, heterogeneous cycle lengths, lack of ovulation timing controls, and oral contraceptive use. Because of these methodological issues and the limited nature of these studies, much remains unknown about premenstrual sleep.

Most women with PMDD seeking psychiatric help for this disorder present with symptoms of premenstrual depression, anxiety, and/or irritability. Several treatment strategies currently exist that target these symptoms and seem to be beneficial in treating them.[33] The selective serotonin-reuptake inhibitors fluoxetine and sertraline have been approved by the US Food and Drug Administration for the treatment of PMDD.

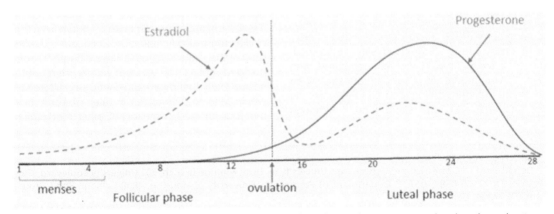

Fig. 1. Changes in estradiol and progesterone across a typical 28-day ovulatory menstrual cycle, where day 1 represents the first day of bleeding. (*From* Baker FC, Lee KA. Menstrual cycle effects on sleep. Sleep Med Clin 2018;13:284; with permission.)

Fluoxetine,[34–37] sertraline,[38] and clomipramine[39,40] seem to be highly effective for treatment of depression; however, few data are available on the safety and efficacy of using selective serotonin-reuptake inhibitors to treat sleep disturbance and insomnia in PMS and PMDD. The evidence for nonpharmacological treatments, such as cognitive behavioral therapy for insomnia (CBT-I) have been summarized in several meta-analyses,[41–43] which led to its recognition as a first-line treatment of insomnia by the NIH Consensus Statement[44] and the American College of Physicians.[45] However, the efficacy of CBT-I in improving sleep and menstrual symptoms has not been examined. It remains unclear if CBT-I is efficacious for women with PMS/PMDD and if special treatment considerations should be made (eg, targeting other PMS symptoms such as menstrual pain[46] or using CBT-I skills intermittently during late luteal phase of a women's menstrual cycle, as is done to treat mood symptoms,[47–49] when symptoms are likely to be the most problematic).

PREGNANCY

Pregnancy brings about significant fluctuations in hormones that affect the sleep-wake cycle and cause physiologic changes that lead to sleep disturbance. In addition to the hormonal changes, pregnancy itself causes a multitude of anatomic and physiologic changes; which are essential to maintain the pregnancy, but can also contribute to sleep problems. Common symptoms, such as anxiety, urinary frequency, backache, fetal movement, general abdominal discomfort, breast tenderness, leg cramps, heart burn, and reflux cause sleep disturbance during pregnancy. Complaints of sleep disturbance during pregnancy generally start at the onset of pregnancy and increase in frequency and duration as the pregnancy progresses because of pregnancy-related anatomic, physiologic, and hormonal changes.[50,51] During the first trimester, women tend to sleep longer and experience greater

daytime sleepiness. Cross-sectional and longitudinal studies that use subjective (self-report) and objective (PSG) measures of sleep have consistently documented increased wake after sleep onset and decreased sleep quality during the first trimester relative to pre-pregnancy.[52,53] During the second trimester, daytime sleepiness improves. During the third trimester there is an increase in sleep disruptions with typically 3 to 5 awakenings per night, more daily naps,[54] diminished daytime alertness, more disturbed dreams,[55] and approximately 21% report disturbed sleep at levels consistent with a diagnosis of insomnia disorder[52,56] (**Fig. 2**). Decreased sleep efficiency, increased wake after sleep onset, increased total sleep time (decreased by third trimester), increased stage 1 and 2 sleep, and decreased rapid eye movement (REM) sleep (during late pregnancy) have been noted by PSG recordings.[57–60] Poor and insufficient sleep during pregnancy is also associated with increased circulating levels of inflammatory markers involved in poor health[61–65] and adverse pregnancy outcomes, including intrauterine growth restriction and preterm delivery.[66–72] During the third trimester of pregnancy, insufficient and poor sleep may place women at increased risk for prolonged labor and cesarean deliveries[73–75] and for having an infant small for gestational age.[76]

For most women, sleep disruptions are caused by factors related to pregnancy, such as frequent need for urination during pregnancy.[56] Some women, however, have difficulties initiating sleep and/or returning to sleep, which may be unrelated to perinatal factors. When sleep disturbances are substantial (occur for 3+ nights per week for a period of 3+ months) and are associated with clinically significant distress or impairment of performance or other aspects of functioning, a diagnosis of insomnia disorder diagnosis is warranted. Insomnia may be experienced as a continuation or exacerbation of insomnia disorder that predates pregnancy or it may develop during pregnancy. The prevalence of sleep disturbance

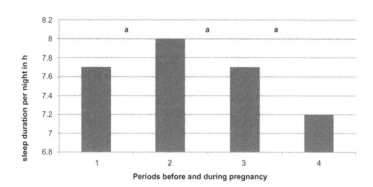

Fig. 2. Evolution of women's sleep duration per night before and during pregnancy. (1) Before pregnancy, (2) first trimester of pregnancy, (3) second trimester of pregnancy, (4) third trimester of pregnancy. ᵃP ≤.001. (*Data from* Bat-Pitault F. Sleep pattern during pregnancy and maternal depression: study of AuBE cohort. J Sleep Disord Manag 2015;1:1.)

among perinatal women is as high as 58%,[77–79] and a probable diagnosis of perinatal insomnia is estimated at 10%.[80] Daytime coping strategies such as napping, spending more time in bed, or increasing caffeine intake can perpetuate sleep difficulties. The presence of insomnia has a significant impact on quality of life and daytime functioning, and its management is imperative.

Pharmacologic treatment of insomnia during pregnancy is typically avoided because of the potential for adverse effects such as low birth weight, preterm deliveries, and cesarean sections in pregnancy.[81–85] Concerns regarding use of sleep medication during pregnancy and lactation make nonpharmacological treatment options for insomnia particularly attractive. CBT-I is a promising intervention for insomnia during pregnancy. A recent study of 187 pregnant women recruited from a low-risk maternity clinic and trade show, revealed that pregnant women preferred CBT-I over pharmacotherapy or acupuncture for treatment of insomnia.[86] Preliminary evidence in an open-pilot trial of 13 pregnant women with insomnia revealed improvements in diary- and actigraphy-assessed sleep onset latency, sleep efficiency, and total sleep time.[87] In addition, symptoms of depression, pregnancy-specific anxiety, and fatigue also improved following treatment.[87] In this trial, CBT-I consisted of 5 weekly 90-minute group sessions and was adapted for pregnant women using the Obesity-Related Behavioral Intervention Trials model[88] from a treatment protocol that was previously validated for oncology patients with comorbid insomnia.[89] The final CBT-I session included a booklet on how to maintain gains in the postpartum period and how to foster optimal infant sleep.[90] Future studies could examine CBT-I tailored further for pregnancy symptoms (eg, overcoming fatigue, strategies to reduce pain/discomfort during pregnancy, minimizing sleep disruption because of urinary frequency at night, increased stress management/relaxation, challenging maladaptive thoughts related to pregnancy and impending labor and delivery, and role transition).

POSTPARTUM

Sleep disturbance during the postpartum period and its effects on maternal role functioning and mother-infant interactions are not well understood. Both self-report and actigraphy studies have demonstrated that nearly 30% of mothers have disturbed sleep after the birth of their baby. The precipitous drop in hormone levels after the birth and unpredictable infant sleep patterns can affect a new mother's sleep. Longitudinal studies have documented that the first 6 months postpartum are associated with a significant increase in wake after sleep onset and a decrease in sleep efficiency compared with the last trimester of pregnancy.[51,60,79,91,92] Fatigue and lack of energy remain high from pregnancy into the postpartum period through the first year after delivery. Sleep begins to normalize around 3 to 6 months postpartum, when infants begin to establish their own circadian rhythm, distinguishing between day and night, and sleep for longer periods of time during the night. Some women may also react to infant waking with catastrophic predictions about the consequences of these disruptions that, in turn, lead to hyperarousal and prolonged wakefulness even after the baby is content and asleep. The response to sleep disruption with distress and urgency to get back to sleep inevitably increase arousal and reduce the likelihood of returning to sleep easily. Other factors such as the mother's age, type of delivery, type of infant feeding, infant temperament, return-to-work issues, prior birth experience, number of other children at home, and availability of nighttime support from the partner or other family member can have an impact on quality and quantity of sleep in new mothers. Many women compensate for their sleep disruptions by spending more time napping during the early postpartum period and going to bed earlier than pre-pregnancy habitual bedtime.[93] Sleep disruptions that may have begun with pregnancy or postpartum-related stressors develop into an insomnia disorder, maintained by maladaptive compensatory behaviors[94] and conditioned hyperarousal.

Negative effects of poor and insufficient sleep during the postpartum period are also associated with mood disturbance and interfere with bonding. Mothers with poorer sleep (lower self-reported sleep quality and a higher number of night waking resulting from infant awakenings) perceived their infants as having lower mood and as being more distressed and tearful.[95] Moreover, insufficient sleep and more time tending to the infant at night predicted poorer maternal-infant attachment. Several studies have documented the relationship between sleep disturbance and subsequent reports of depressive symptoms at a later time among perinatal women (later in pregnancy[96–98] or in the early postpartum[97,99–102]). The association between poor sleep and subsequent depressive symptoms also holds when sleep disturbance is experienced during the early postpartum period, and postpartum depression develops at a later postpartum time.[103–105]

Interventions to improve maternal sleep and fatigue are limited, perhaps because of the universal nature of the experience and the belief that disturbed sleep is an unavoidable part of motherhood. In general, pharmacologic interventions are seldom used in postpartum women who are breastfeeding. Even for women who are not breastfeeding, many choose not to take sedatives or other pharmacologic options because of the need to have a more flexible sleep schedule for infant care. Therefore, behavioral interventions are the primary treatment options. Two pilot studies provide preliminary evidence for the efficacy of CBT-I for postpartum insomnia and both studies demonstrated that the benefits of CBT-I extended beyond improvement in sleep to other domains. One study provided 5 CBT-I sessions, between the second and seventh postpartum weeks, to women who stopped smoking during pregnancy and found a significant decrease in time awake in the middle of the night and a significant increase in nocturnal (as well as per 24 h) sleep time. Importantly, compared with women who did not receive the sleep intervention, those who did undergo CBT-I had lower average daily cigarettes smoked and higher percent cigarette-free days.[106] The second study provided CBT-I to women with postpartum depression who also had disturbed sleep and reported pre- to posttreatment improvement in insomnia severity, sleep quality, sleep efficiency (percent time asleep relative to time in bed), mood, and daytime fatigue.[107] In addition, several randomized controlled trials have evaluated interventions promoting infant sleep by providing education and training on infant sleep strategies to limit the development of unwanted sleep associations, increase the infant's ability to self soothe, and recommend environmental modifications to consolidate infant sleep at night. These trails demonstrated longer and more consolidated sleep periods compared with infants in control conditions.[108–110] Future studies examining CBT-I across pregnancy and into the postpartum period and combining interventions for maternal and infant sleep are still needed. Future studies and interventions could also include the impact of partners or significant others to enhance support for maternal sleep and nighttime parenting responsibilities.

MENOPAUSE

Menopause is a natural process that occurs in women's lives as part of normal aging. Menopause is defined as the cessation of menstruation because of degeneration of ovaries and follicles accompanied by changing ovarian hormone levels (estrogen and progesterone). The World Health Organization[111] characterizes menopause as the permanent cessation of menstrual periods that occurs naturally or is induced by surgery, chemotherapy, or radiation. More recently menopause has been categorized in stages such as menopausal transition (defined by standardized criteria[112] as variable cycle length 7 days different from the normal cycle or >2 skipped cycles and an interval of amenorrhea of 2–12 months) or postmenopausal (defined as >12 months since last menstrual period) (**Fig. 3**). Menopause occurs between 50 and 52 years of age for Western women, but the range can vary based on race and ethnicity as well as lifestyle factors.[113] The worldwide population of 470 million postmenopausal women is expected to increase, as 1.5 million women enter menopause each year, reaching a total of 1.2 billion by the year 2030.[111] Most women now live long enough to become menopausal and can expect to live at least another 30 years beyond their final menstrual period.

Many women go through the menopausal transition with few or no symptoms, whereas a small percentage of women suffer from symptoms severe enough to interfere with their ability to function effectively at home, work, or school. Common complaints include hot flashes, night sweats, insomnia, mood changes, fatigue, and excessive daytime sleepiness. In the 2005 NIH State-of-the-Science Conference panel report on menopause-related symptoms, sleep disturbance was identified as a core symptom of menopause.[114] The prevalence of insomnia, defined as disturbed sleep associated with distress or impairment, is estimated at 38% to 60% in peri- and postmenopausal women.[114–116] Troubled sleep was reported by 54% to 58% of women between 40 and 60 years of age in the Ohio Midlife Women's study.[117] The Wisconsin Sleep Cohort found that perimenopausal women and postmenopausal women were twice as likely to be dissatisfied with their sleep as premenopausal women.[118] The Study of Women's Health Across the Nation has shown that difficulty sleeping is reported by 38% of women between 40 and 55 years of age, with higher levels among late perimenopausal (45.4%) and surgical postmenopausal (47.6%) women.[116]

The prevalence on nocturnal hot flashes/night sweats is generally believed to occur in 60% to 80% of women during the menopausal transition[119] and persist for 4 to 5 years on average.[120,121] When hot flashes occur during the night, they frequently awaken women from sleep; although not every nocturnal flash is associated with an awakening. Women with nocturnal flashes may also experience awakenings that are unrelated to a vasomotor event. Indeed, insomnia can occur during menopause independent of nocturnal flashes. Although self-reported

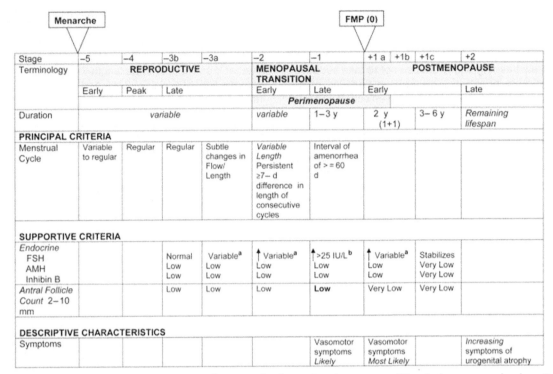

Menarche						FMP (0)			

Stage	−5	−4	−3b	−3a	−2	−1	+1a	+1b	+1c	+2
Terminology	REPRODUCTIVE				MENOPAUSAL TRANSITION		POSTMENOPAUSE			
	Early	Peak	Late		Early	Late	Early			Late
					Perimenopause					
Duration	variable				variable	1–3 y	2 y (1+1)		3–6 y	Remaining lifespan
PRINCIPAL CRITERIA										
Menstrual Cycle	Variable to regular	Regular	Regular	Subtle changes in Flow/ Length	Variable Length Persistent ≥7– d difference in length of consecutive cycles	Interval of amenorrhea of > = 60 d				
SUPPORTIVE CRITERIA										
Endocrine FSH AMH Inhibin B			Normal Low Low	Variable[a] Low Low	↑ Variable[a] Low Low	↑ >25 IU/L[b] Low Low	↑ Variable[a] Low Low	Stabilizes Very Low Very Low		
Antral Follicle Count 2–10 mm			Low	Low	Low	**Low**	Very Low	Very Low		
DESCRIPTIVE CHARACTERISTICS										
Symptoms					Vasomotor symptoms Likely	Vasomotor symptoms Most Likely				Increasing symptoms of urogenital atrophy

Fig. 3. The STRAW+10 staging system for reproductive aging in women. [a]Blood draw on cycle days 2 to 5 = elevated. [b]Approximate expected level based on assays using current pituitary standard.[67–69] (*From* Harlow SD, Gass M, Hall JE, et al. Executive summary of the Stages of Reproductive Aging Workshop+10: addressing the unfinished agenda of staging reproductive aging. Climacteric 2012;15(2):105–14; with permission.)

nocturnal flashes correlate with poor subjective sleep quality, such association is less clear when objective sleep measures are used.[118,122,123] There is only limited and contradictory evidence supporting an association between nocturnal flashes and sleep disturbance when both variables were measured objectively.[118,122–128] This may be, in part, due to the stage of sleep during which hot flashes are occurring. When taking sleep stage into account, several studies have demonstrated a relatively low incidence of hot flashes during REM sleep, which has been postulated to be because of the inhibition of thermoregulatory responses during REM sleep.[129] Contradictory evidence may also be due to the way in which investigators characterized hot flashes associated with awakenings, and the duration of the window for detecting an awakening before or after the hot flash occurred.

Vasomotor symptoms, including nocturnal hot flashes and night sweats, may be a precipitating factor in the development of insomnia, but physiologic arousals, behavioral conditioning, and misguided coping attempts seem to prolong insomnia.[130] CBT-I targets these behaviors and has been shown to be efficacious for the treatment of chronic insomnia in randomized trials of older adults[131] and for midlife women.[132–134] Telephone-delivered CBT-I has recently been evaluated for insomnia during the menopausal transition in a randomized clinical trial of peri- and postmenopausal women with insomnia symptoms as well as daily hot flashes.[134,135] Compared with a menopause education control condition, 8 weeks of telephone-delivered CBT-I led to a greater reduction in insomnia symptoms, with improvements maintained at 6 months posttreatment.[134] Another randomized clinical trial of 150 postmenopausal women with insomnia were randomized to 1 of 3 conditions: face-to-face CBT-I, sleep restriction only, or sleep hygiene education control. The investigators found that the participants treated with CBT-I had a decrease in the insomnia severity index by 7.7 points, sleep restriction by 6.5 points, and sleep hygiene control by 1.1 points. Participants who received CBT-I were generally more likely to remit than participants who received sleep restriction alone.[133] These studies have examined traditional CBT-I or sleep restriction component of CBT-I in midlife women.

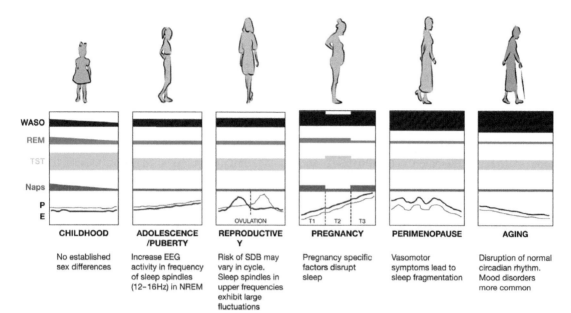

Fig. 4. Sleep in women across the lifespan. E, estrogen; NREM, non-rapid eye movement; P, progesterone; REM, rapid eye movement; SDB, sleep-disordered breathing; T, trimester; TST, total sleep time; WASO, wake after sleep onset. (*From* Pengo MF, Won CH, Bourjeily G. Sleep in women across the life span. Chest 2018;154(1):196–206; with permission.)

By focusing on distress following the hot flash experience, the principles of CBT can also be used to reduce suffering from hot flashes. Psychological factors, such as reaction to stress, seem to play a role; with past findings that higher levels of perceived control and lower distress were associated with fewer hot flashes.[136–138] Women who perceive greater control over their reactions to hot flashes tend to regard their flashes as less problematic and report fewer hot flashes[137] This suggests that addressing reactions to hot flashes and providing strategies for coping with hot flashes could reduce distress associated with hot flashes. Indeed, several studies have provided empirical support demonstrating CBT as an effective strategy for coping with hot flashes and other menopausal symptoms.[139–146] Future studies combining CBT for insomnia and hot flashes could prove to be beneficial for women bothered by multiple symptoms during menopause, including insomnia and hot flashes.

SUMMARY

Sleep disturbances and disorders are common across a woman's lifespan. Important biological events, often mediated by hormones and physiologic changes, such as menstruation, pregnancy, and menopause commonly affect and often cause dissatisfaction with sleep (**Fig. 4**).

Given that the negative effects of poor sleep extend beyond tiredness and fatigue but also impair daytime functioning and mood, identification and treatment of these disorders is vital to a woman's quality of life. Women looking to treat their sleep problems have many options. Nonpharmacological treatments, such as CBT-I, offer longer-lasting improvements for insomnia without the side-effects that often accompany medications.

Despite advancing research in sleep and women's health, there are several areas that deserve more focused research. In studies examining sex differences, the menstrual phase should be considered and documented. Whereas it is known that the hormones are linked to sleep and that the variability across the menstrual cycle causes changes in sleep quality, there are few studies that have explored insomnia treatment options in women with PMS and PMDD and the interaction of sleep and mood disturbances and menstrual pain. There are a greater number of published studies examining CBT-I in perinatal and perimenopausal women. However, few studies have tailored CBT-I to multiple symptoms women may be experiencing. In addition, the high prevalence of women experiencing insomnia during times of reproductive hormonal change relative to the low number of trained providers able to effectively deliver CBT-I remains unbalanced.[147] Thus, future research should focus on dissemination and implementation of CBT-I to improve access to care, with particular attention on using health technologies to reach more patients. Examining the effectiveness of CBT-I and its downstream effects on immune functioning, chronic health conditions, and recovery is also greatly needed.

ACKNOWLEGMENT

This work was supported by the National Institutes of Nursing Research (R01NR018342 and K23NR014008 to S.N.).

REFERENCES

1. Akerstedt T, Knutsson A, Westerholm P, et al. Sleep disturbances, work stress and work hours: a cross-sectional study. J Psychosom Res 2002;53(3):741–8.
2. Lindberg E, Janson C, Gislason T, et al. Sleep disturbances in a young adult population: can gender differences be explained by differences in psychological status? Sleep 1997;20(6):381–7.
3. Jaussent I, Dauvilliers Y, Ancelin ML, et al. Insomnia symptoms in older adults: associated factors and gender differences. Am J Geriatr Psychiatry 2011;19(1):88–97.
4. Singareddy R, Vgontzas AN, Fernandez-Mendoza J, et al. Risk factors for incident chronic insomnia: a general population prospective study. Sleep Med 2012;13(4):346–53.
5. Baker FC, Wolfson AR, Lee KA. Association of sociodemographic, lifestyle, and health factors with sleep quality and daytime sleepiness in women: findings from the 2007 National Sleep Foundation "Sleep in America Poll". J Womens Health (Larchmt) 2009;18(6):841–9.
6. Ferguson KA, Ono T, Lowe AA, et al. The relationship between obesity and craniofacial structure in obstructive sleep apnea. Chest 1995;108(2):375–81.
7. Carrier J, Land S, Buysse DJ, et al. The effects of age and gender on sleep EEG power spectral density in the middle years of life (ages 20–60 years old). Psychophysiology 2001;38(2):232–42.
8. Bixler EO, Papaliaga MN, Vgontzas AN, et al. Women sleep objectively better than men and the sleep of young women is more resilient to external stressors: effects of age and menopause. J Sleep Res 2009;18(2):221–8.
9. Jean-Louis G, Mendlowicz MV, Von Gizycki H, et al. Assessment of physical activity and sleep by actigraphy: examination of gender differences. J Womens Health Gend Based Med 1999;8(8):1113–7.
10. Rediehs MH, Reis JS, Creason NS. Sleep in old age: focus on gender differences. Sleep 1990;13(5):410–24.
11. Driver HS, Baker FC. Menstrual factors in sleep. Sleep Med Rev 1998;2(4):213–29.
12. Halbreich U, Borenstein J, Pearlstein T, et al. The prevalence, impairment, impact, and burden of premenstrual dysphoric disorder (PMS/PMDD). Psychoneuroendocrinology 2003;28(Suppl 3):1–23.
13. Halbreich U, Backstrom T, Eriksson E, et al. Clinical diagnostic criteria for premenstrual syndrome and guidelines for their quantification for research studies. Gynecol Endocrinol 2007;23(3):123–30.
14. de Carvalho AB, Cardoso TA, Mondin TC, et al. Prevalence and factors associated with premenstrual dysphoric disorder: a community sample of young adult women. Psychiatry Res 2018;268:42–5.
15. Khazaie H, Ghadami MR, Khaledi-Paveh B, et al. Sleep quality in university students with premenstrual dysphoric disorder. Shanghai Arch Psychiatry 2016;28(3):131–8.
16. Liu X, Chen H, Liu ZZ, et al. Early menarche and menstrual problems are associated with sleep disturbance in a large sample of Chinese adolescent girls. Sleep 2017;40(9). https://doi.org/10.1093/sleep/zsx107.
17. Kim T, Nam GE, Han B, et al. Associations of mental health and sleep duration with menstrual cycle irregularity: a population-based study. Arch Womens Ment Health 2018. https://doi.org/10.1007/s00737-018-0872-8.
18. Kang W, Jang KH, Lim HM, et al. The menstrual cycle associated with insomnia in newly employed nurses performing shift work: a 12-month follow-up study. Int Arch Occup Environ Health 2019;92(2):227–35.
19. Baker FC, Driver HS. Self-reported sleep across the menstrual cycle in young, healthy women. J Psychosom Res 2004;56(2):239–43.
20. Cohen LS, Soares CN, Otto MW, et al. Prevalence and predictors of premenstrual dysphoric disorder (PMDD) in older premenopausal women. The Harvard Study of Moods and Cycles. J Affect Disord 2002;70(2):125–32.
21. Hachul H, Andersen ML, Bittencourt LR, et al. Does the reproductive cycle influence sleep patterns in women with sleep complaints? Climacteric 2010;13(6):594–603.
22. Lamarche LJ, Driver HS, Wiebe S, et al. Nocturnal sleep, daytime sleepiness, and napping among women with significant emotional/behavioral premenstrual symptoms. J Sleep Res 2007;16(3):262–8.
23. Smith MJ, Schmidt PJ, Rubinow DR. Operationalizing DSM-IV criteria for PMDD: selecting symptomatic and asymptomatic cycles for research. J Psychiatr Res 2003;37(1):75–83.
24. Woosley JA, Lichstein KL. Dysmenorrhea, the menstrual cycle, and sleep. Behav Med 2014;40(1):14–21.

25. Lee KA, Baker FC, Newton KM, et al. The Influence of reproductive status and age on women's sleep. J Womens Health (larchmt) 2008;17(7):1209–14.

26. Moline ML, Broch L, Zak R. Sleep in women across the life cycle from adulthood through menopause. Med Clin North Am 2004;88(3):705–36, ix.

27. Schmidt PJ, Martinez PE, Nieman LK, et al. Premenstrual dysphoric disorder symptoms following ovarian suppression: triggered by change in ovarian steroid levels but not continuous stable levels. Am J Psychiatry 2017;174(10):980–9.

28. Zheng H, Harlow SD, Kravitz HM, et al. Actigraphy-defined measures of sleep and movement across the menstrual cycle in midlife menstruating women: study of women's health across the nation sleep study. Menopause 2015;22(1):66–74.

29. Baker FC, Kahan TL, Trinder J, et al. Sleep quality and the sleep electroencephalogram in women with severe premenstrual syndrome. Sleep 2007; 30(10):1283–91.

30. Baker FC, Sassoon SA, Kahan T, et al. Perceived poor sleep quality in the absence of polysomnographic sleep disturbance in women with severe premenstrual syndrome. J Sleep Res 2012;21(5): 535–45.

31. Parry BL, Mostofi N, LeVeau B, et al. Sleep EEG studies during early and late partial sleep deprivation in premenstrual dysphoric disorder and normal control subjects. Psychiatry Res 1999;85(2): 127–43.

32. Sharkey KM, Crawford SL, Kim S, et al. Objective sleep interruption and reproductive hormone dynamics in the menstrual cycle. Sleep Med 2014; 15(6):688–93.

33. Altshuler LL, Hendrick V, Parry B. Pharmacological management of premenstrual disorder. Harv Rev Psychiatry 1995;2(5):233–45.

34. Menkes DB, Taghavi E, Mason PA, et al. Fluoxetine treatment of severe premenstrual syndrome. BMJ 1992;305(6849):346–7.

35. Steiner M, Steinberg S, Stewart D, et al. Fluoxetine in the treatment of premenstrual dysphoria. Canadian Fluoxetine/Premenstrual Dysphoria Collaborative Study Group. N Engl J Med 1995;332(23): 1529–34.

36. Stone AB, Pearlstein TB, Brown WA. Fluoxetine in the treatment of late luteal phase dysphoric disorder. J Clin Psychiatry 1991;52(7):290–3.

37. Wood SH, Mortola JF, Chan YF, et al. Treatment of premenstrual syndrome with fluoxetine: a double-blind, placebo-controlled, crossover study. Obstet Gynecol 1992;80(3 Pt 1):339–44.

38. Yonkers KA, Halbreich U, Freeman E, et al. Symptomatic improvement of premenstrual dysphoric disorder with sertraline treatment. A randomized controlled trial. Sertraline Premenstrual Dysphoric Collaborative Study Group. JAMA 1997;278(12): 983–8.

39. Sundblad C, Modigh K, Andersch B, et al. Clomipramine effectively reduces premenstrual irritability and dysphoria: a placebo-controlled trial. Acta Psychiatr Scand 1992;85(1):39–47.

40. Sundblad C, Hedberg MA, Eriksson E. Clomipramine administered during the luteal phase reduces the symptoms of premenstrual syndrome: a placebo-controlled trial. Neuropsychopharmacology 1993;9(2):133–45.

41. Morin CM, Culbert JP, Schwartz SM. Nonpharmacological interventions for insomnia: a meta-analysis of treatment efficacy. Am J Psychiatry 1994;151(8):1172–80.

42. Murtagh DR, Greenwood KM. Identifying effective psychological treatments for insomnia: a meta-analysis. J Consult Clin Psychol 1995;63(1):79–89.

43. Smith MT, Perlis ML, Park A, et al. Comparative meta-analysis of pharmacotherapy and behavior therapy for persistent insomnia. Am J Psychiatry 2002;159(1):5–11.

44. National Institutes of Health. National Institutes of Health State of the Science Conference statement on Manifestations and Management of Chronic Insomnia in Adults, June 13–15, 2005. Sleep 2005;28(9):1049–57.

45. Qaseem A, Kansagara D, Forciea MA, et al. Management of chronic insomnia disorder in adults: a clinical practice guideline from the American College of Physicians. Ann Intern Med 2016;165(2): 125–33.

46. Araujo P, Hachul H, Santos-Silva R, et al. Sleep pattern in women with menstrual pain. Sleep Med 2011;12(10):1028–30.

47. Freeman EW, Rickels K, Sondheimer SJ, et al. Continuous or intermittent dosing with sertraline for patients with severe premenstrual syndrome or premenstrual dysphoric disorder. Am J Psychiatry 2004;161(2):343–51.

48. Halbreich U, Bergeron R, Yonkers KA, et al. Efficacy of intermittent, luteal phase sertraline treatment of premenstrual dysphoric disorder. Obstet Gynecol 2002;100(6):1219–29.

49. Kornstein SG, Pearlstein TB, Fayyad R, et al. Low-dose sertraline in the treatment of moderate-to-severe premenstrual syndrome: efficacy of 3 dosing strategies. J Clin Psychiatry 2006;67(10):1624–32.

50. Little SE, McNamara CJ, Miller RC. Sleep changes in normal pregnancy. Obstet Gynecol 2014; 123(Suppl 1):153S.

51. Hertz G, Fast A, Feinsilver SH, et al. Sleep in normal late pregnancy. Sleep 1992;15(3):246–51.

52. Hedman C, Pohjasvaara T, Tolonen U, et al. Effects of pregnancy on mothers' sleep. Sleep Med 2002; 3(1):37–42.

53. Santiago JR, Nolledo MS, Kinzler W, et al. Sleep and sleep disorders in pregnancy. Ann Intern Med 2001;134(5):396–408.

54. Tsai SY, Lin JW, Kuo LT, et al. Daily sleep and fatigue characteristics in nulliparous women during the third trimester of pregnancy. Sleep 2012; 35(2):257–62.

55. Lara-Carrasco J, Simard V, Saint-Onge K, et al. Disturbed dreaming during the third trimester of pregnancy. Sleep Med 2014;15(6):694–700.

56. Baratte-Beebe KR, Lee K. Sources of midsleep awakenings in childbearing women. Clin Nurs Res 1999;8(4):386–97.

57. Kizilirmak A, Timur S, Kartal B. Insomnia in pregnancy and factors related to insomnia. ScientificWorldJournal 2012;2012:197093.

58. Driver HS, Shapiro CM. A longitudinal study of sleep stages in young women during pregnancy and postpartum. Sleep 1992;15(5):449–53.

59. Pien GW, Schwab RJ. Sleep disorders during pregnancy. Sleep 2004;27(7):1405–17.

60. Lee KA, Zaffke ME, McEnany G. Parity and sleep patterns during and after pregnancy. Obstet Gynecol 2000;95(1):14–8.

61. von Kanel R, Dimsdale JE, Ancoli-Israel S, et al. Poor sleep is associated with higher plasma proinflammatory cytokine interleukin-6 and procoagulant marker fibrin D-dimer in older caregivers of people with Alzheimer's disease. J Am Geriatr Soc 2006;54(3):431–7.

62. Vgontzas AN, Zoumakis E, Bixler EO, et al. Adverse effects of modest sleep restriction on sleepiness, performance, and inflammatory cytokines. J Clin Endocrinol Metab 2004;89(5):2119–26.

63. McDade TW, Hawkley LC, Cacioppo JT. Psychosocial and behavioral predictors of inflammation in middle-aged and older adults: the Chicago Health, Aging, and Social Relations Study. Psychosom Med 2006;68(3):376–81.

64. Meier-Ewert HK, Ridker PM, Rifai N, et al. Effect of sleep loss on C-reactive protein, an inflammatory marker of cardiovascular risk. J Am Coll Cardiol 2004;43(4):678–83.

65. Irwin MR, Wang M, Campomayor CO, et al. Sleep deprivation and activation of morning levels of cellular and genomic markers of inflammation. Arch Intern Med 2006;166(16):1756–62.

66. Dudley D. Cytokines in preterm and term parturition. In: Hill J, editor. Cytokines in human reproduction. New York: John Wiley & Sons, Inc.; 2000. p. 171–202.

67. Holst RM, Mattsby-Baltzer I, Wennerholm UB, et al. Interleukin-6 and interleukin-8 in cervical fluid in a population of Swedish women in preterm labor: relationship to microbial invasion of the amniotic fluid, intra-amniotic inflammation, and preterm delivery. Acta Obstet Gynecol Scand 2005;84(6):551–7.

68. Menon R, Merialdi M, Lombardi SJ, et al. Differences in the placental membrane cytokine response: a possible explanation for the racial disparity in preterm birth. Am J Reprod Immunol 2006;56(2):112–8.

69. Vogel I, Thorsen P, Curry A, et al. Biomarkers for the prediction of preterm delivery. Acta Obstet Gynecol Scand 2005;84(6):516–25.

70. Bartha JL, Romero-Carmona R, Comino-Delgado R. Inflammatory cytokines in intrauterine growth retardation. Acta Obstet Gynecol Scand 2003;82(12):1099–102.

71. Holcberg G, Huleihel M, Sapir O, et al. Increased production of tumor necrosis factor-alpha TNF-alpha by IUGR human placentae. Eur J Obstet Gynecol Reprod Biol 2001;94(1):69–72.

72. Romero R, Espinoza J, Goncalves LF, et al. Inflammation in preterm and term labour and delivery. Semin Fetal Neonatal Med 2006;11(5):317–26.

73. Lee KA, Gay CL. Sleep in late pregnancy predicts length of labor and type of delivery. Am J Obstet Gynecol 2004;191(6):2041–6.

74. Okun ML, Roberts JM, Marsland AL, et al. How disturbed sleep may be a risk factor for adverse pregnancy outcomes. Obstet Gynecol Surv 2009; 64(4):273–80.

75. Okun ML, Luther JF, Wisniewski SR, et al. Disturbed sleep, a novel risk factor for preterm birth? J Womens Health (Larchmt) 2012;21(1): 54–60.

76. Chang J, Chien L, Duntley S, et al. Sleep duration during pregnancy and maternal and fetal outcomes: a pilot study using actigraphy. Sleep 2011;34(Suppl):A317.

77. Dorheim SK, Bondevik GT, Eberhard-Gran M, et al. Sleep and depression in postpartum women: a population-based study. Sleep 2009; 32(7):847–55.

78. Swanson LM, Pickett SM, Flynn H, et al. Relationships among depression, anxiety, and insomnia symptoms in perinatal women seeking mental health treatment. J Womens Health (Larchmt) 2011;20(4):553–8.

79. Mindell JA, Jacobson BJ. Sleep disturbances during pregnancy. J Obstet Gynecol Neonatal Nurs 2000;29(6):590–7.

80. Manber R, Steidtmann D, Chambers AS, et al. Factors associated with clinically significant insomnia among pregnant low-income Latinas. J Womens Health (Larchmt) 2013;22(8):694–701.

81. Okun ML, Ebert R, Saini B. A review of sleep-promoting medications used in pregnancy. Am J Obstet Gynecol 2015;212(4):428–41.

82. Wang LH, Lin HC, Lin CC, et al. Increased risk of adverse pregnancy outcomes in women receiving zolpidem during pregnancy. Clin Pharmacol Ther 2010;88(3):369–74.

83. Ibrahim S, Foldvary-Schaefer N. Sleep disorders in pregnancy: implications, evaluation, and treatment. Neurol Clin 2012;30(3):925–36.
84. McLafferty LP, Spada M, Gopalan P. Pharmacologic treatment of sleep disorders in pregnancy. Sleep Med Clin 2018;13(2):243–50.
85. Zammit G. Comparative tolerability of newer agents for insomnia. Drug Saf 2009;32(9):735–48.
86. Sedov ID, Goodman SH, Tomfohr-Madsen LM. Insomnia treatment preferences during pregnancy. J Obstet Gynecol neonatal Nurs 2017;46(3):e95–104.
87. Tomfohr-Madsen LM, Clayborne ZM, Rouleau CR, et al. Sleeping for two: an open-pilot study of cognitive behavioral therapy for insomnia in pregnancy. Behav Sleep Med 2017;15(5):377–93.
88. Czajkowski SM, Powell LH, Adler N, et al. From ideas to efficacy: the ORBIT model for developing behavioral treatments for chronic diseases. Health Psychol 2015;34(10):971–82.
89. Garland SN, Carlson LE, Stephens AJ, et al. Mindfulness-based stress reduction compared with cognitive behavioral therapy for the treatment of insomnia comorbid with cancer: a randomized, partially blinded, noninferiority trial. J Clin Oncol 2014;32(5):449–57.
90. Stremler R, Hodnett E, Kenton L, et al. Effect of behavioural-educational intervention on sleep for primiparous women and their infants in early postpartum: multisite randomised controlled trial. BMJ 2013;346:f1164.
91. Montgomery-Downs HE, Insana SP, Clegg-Kraynok MM, et al. Normative longitudinal maternal sleep: the first 4 postpartum months. Am J Obstet Gynecol 2010;203(5):465.e1-7.
92. Brunner DP, Munch M, Biedermann K, et al. Changes in sleep and sleep electroencephalogram during pregnancy. Sleep 1994;17(7):576–82.
93. Swain AM, O'Hara MW, Starr KR, et al. A prospective study of sleep, mood, and cognitive function in postpartum and nonpostpartum women. Obstet Gynecol 1997;90(3):381–6.
94. Spielman AJ, Caruso LS, Glovinsky PB. A behavioral perspective on insomnia treatment. Psychiatr Clin North Am 1987;10(4):541–53.
95. Tikotzky L, Chambers AS, Gaylor E, et al. Maternal sleep and depressive symptoms: links with infant negative affectivity. Infant Behav Dev 2010;33(4):605–12.
96. Skouteris H, Germano C, Wertheim EH, et al. Sleep quality and depression during pregnancy: a prospective study. J Sleep Res 2008;17(2):217–20.
97. Park EM, Meltzer-Brody S, Stickgold R. Poor sleep maintenance and subjective sleep quality are associated with postpartum maternal depression symptom severity. Arch Womens Ment Health 2013;16(6):539–47.
98. Kamysheva E, Skouteris H, Wertheim EH, et al. A prospective investigation of the relationships among sleep quality, physical symptoms, and depressive symptoms during pregnancy. J Affect Disord 2010;123(1–3):317–20.
99. Dorheim SK, Bjorvatn B, Eberhard-Gran M. Can insomnia in pregnancy predict postpartum depression? A longitudinal, population-based study. PLoS One 2014;9(4):e94674.
100. Wolfson AR, Crowley SJ, Anwer U, et al. Changes in sleep patterns and depressive symptoms in first-time mothers: last trimester to 1-year postpartum. Behav Sleep Med 2003;1(1):54–67.
101. Bei B, Milgrom J, Ericksen J, et al. Subjective perception of sleep, but not its objective quality, is associated with immediate postpartum mood disturbances in healthy women. Sleep 2010;33(4):531–8.
102. Wilkie G, Shapiro CM. Sleep deprivation and the postnatal blues. J Psychosom Res 1992;36(4):309–16.
103. Doering J, Szabo A. Sleep quality and depression symptoms in disadvantaged postpartum women. Sleep 2011;34:A319.
104. Okun ML, Luther J, Prather AA, et al. Changes in sleep quality, but not hormones predict time to postpartum depression recurrence. J Affect Disord 2011;130(3):378–84.
105. Tsai SY, Thomas KA. Sleep disturbances and depressive symptoms in healthy postpartum women: a pilot study. Res Nurs Health 2012;35(3):314–23.
106. Stone K. Effects of a behavioral sleep intervention on postpartum sleep. Sleep 2011;34:A320.
107. Swanson L, Arnedt J, Adams J, et al. An open pilot of cognitive behavioral therapy for insomnia in women with postpartum depression. Sleep 2011;34:A319.
108. St James-Roberts I, Sleep J, Morris S, et al. Use of a behavioural programme in the first 3 months to prevent infant crying and sleeping problems. J Paediatr Child Health 2001;37(3):289–97.
109. Symon BG, Marley JE, Martin AJ, et al. Effect of a consultation teaching behaviour modification on sleep performance in infants: a randomised controlled trial. Med J Aust 2005;182(5):215–8.
110. Wolfson A, Lacks P, Futterman A. Effects of parent training on infant sleeping patterns, parents' stress, and perceived parental competence. J Consult Clin Psychol 1992;60(1):41–8.
111. WHO. Research on the menopause in the 1990s. WHO; 1996.
112. Soules MR, Sherman S, Parrott E, et al. Executive summary: stages of reproductive aging workshop (STRAW). Climacteric 2001;4(4):267–72.
113. Gold EB. The timing of the age at which natural menopause occurs. Obstet Gynecol Clin North Am 2011;38(3):425–40.

114. National Institutes of Health. National Institutes of Health State-of-the-Science Conference statement: management of menopause-related symptoms. Ann Intern Med 2005;142(12 Pt 1):1003–13.

115. Kravitz HM, Ganz PA, Bromberger J, et al. Sleep difficulty in women at midlife: a community survey of sleep and the menopausal transition. Menopause 2003;10(1):19–28.

116. Kravitz HM, Zhao X, Bromberger JT, et al. Sleep disturbance during the menopausal transition in a multi-ethnic community sample of women. Sleep 2008;31(7):979–90.

117. Glazer G, Zeller R, Delumba L, et al. The Ohio Midlife Women's Study. Health Care Women Int 2002;23(6–7):612–30.

118. Young T, Rabago D, Zgierska A, et al. Objective and subjective sleep quality in premenopausal, perimenopausal, and postmenopausal women in the Wisconsin Sleep Cohort Study. Sleep 2003; 26(6):667–72.

119. Gold EB, Sternfeld B, Kelsey JL, et al. Relation of demographic and lifestyle factors to symptoms in a multi-racial/ethnic population of women 40–55 years of age. Am J Epidemiol 2000;152(5):463–73.

120. Col NF, Guthrie JR, Politi M, et al. Duration of vasomotor symptoms in middle-aged women: a longitudinal study. Menopause 2009;16(3):453–7.

121. Politi MC, Schleinitz MD, Col NF. Revisiting the duration of vasomotor symptoms of menopause: a meta-analysis. J Gen Intern Med 2008;23(9):1507–13.

122. Shaver J, Giblin E, Lentz M, et al. Sleep patterns and stability in perimenopausal women. Sleep 1988;11(6):556–61.

123. Ensrud KE, Stone KL, Blackwell TL, et al. Frequency and severity of hot flashes and sleep disturbance in postmenopausal women with hot flashes. Menopause 2009;16(2):286–92.

124. Savard J, Davidson JR, Ivers H, et al. The association between nocturnal hot flashes and sleep in breast cancer survivors. J Pain Symptom Manage 2004;27(6):513–22.

125. Freedman RR, Roehrs TA. Lack of sleep disturbance from menopausal hot flashes. Fertil Steril 2004;82(1):138–44.

126. Erlik Y, Tataryn IV, Meldrum DR, et al. Association of waking episodes with menopausal hot flushes. JAMA 1981;245(17):1741–4.

127. Freedman RR, Benton MD, Genik RJ 2nd, et al. Cortical activation during menopausal hot flashes. Fertil Steril 2006;85(3):674–8.

128. Woodward S, Freedman RR. The thermoregulatory effects of menopausal hot flashes on sleep. Sleep 1994;17(6):497–501.

129. Freedman RR, Roehrs TA. Effects of REM sleep and ambient temperature on hot flash-induced sleep disturbance. Menopause 2006;13(4): 576–83.

130. Krystal AD, Edinger J, Wohlgemuth W, et al. Sleep in peri-menopausal and post-menopausal women. Sleep Med Rev 1998;2(4):243–53.

131. Sivertsen B, Omvik S, Pallesen S, et al. Cognitive behavioral therapy vs zopiclone for treatment of chronic primary insomnia in older adults: a randomized controlled trial. JAMA 2006;295(24): 2851–8.

132. Arnedt JT, Cuddihy L, Swanson LM, et al. Randomized controlled trial of telephone-delivered cognitive behavioral therapy for chronic insomnia. Sleep 2013;36(3):353–62.

133. Drake CL, Kalmbach DA, Arnedt JT, et al. Treating chronic insomnia in postmenopausal women: a randomized clinical trial comparing cognitive-behavioral therapy for insomnia (CBTI), Sleep restriction therapy, and sleep hygiene education. Sleep 2018. https://doi.org/10.1093/sleep/zsy217.

134. McCurry SM, Guthrie KA, Morin CM, et al. Telephone-based cognitive behavioral therapy for insomnia in perimenopausal and postmenopausal women with vasomotor symptoms: a MsFLASH randomized clinical trial. JAMA Intern Med 2016; 176(7):913–20.

135. Guthrie KA, Larson JC, Ensrud KE, et al. Effects of pharmacologic and nonpharmacologic interventions on insomnia symptoms and self-reported sleep quality in women with hot flashes: a pooled analysis of individual participant data from four MsFLASH trials. Sleep 2018;41(1). https://doi.org/10.1093/sleep/zsx190.

136. Hunter MS, Liao KL. A psychological analysis of menopausal hot flushes. Br J Clin Psychol 1995; 34(Pt 4):589–99.

137. Reynolds FA. Perceived control over menopausal hot flushes: exploring the correlates of a standardised measure. Maturitas 1997;27(3): 215–21.

138. Hunter MS, Mann E. A cognitive model of menopausal hot flushes and night sweats. J Psychosom Res 2010;69(5):491–501.

139. Adler JEBK, Armbruster U, Decio R, et al. Cognitive-behavioural group intervention for climacteric syndrome. Psychother Psychosom 2006;75(5): 298–303.

140. Atema V, van Leeuwen M, Oldenburg HSA, et al. An internet-based cognitive behavioral therapy for treatment-induced menopausal symptoms in breast cancer survivors: results of a pilot study. Menopause 2017;24(7):762–7.

141. Smith M, in Collaboration with the British Menopause Society. Cognitive behaviour therapy (CBT) for menopausal symptoms: information for GPs and health professionals. Post Reprod Health 2017;23(2):83–4.

142. Stefanopoulou E, Grunfeld EA. Mind-body interventions for vasomotor symptoms in healthy

menopausal women and breast cancer survivors. A systematic review. J Psychosom Obstet Gynaecol 2017;38(3):210–25.

143. Hunter MS, Hardy C, Norton S, et al. Study protocol of a multicentre randomised controlled trial of self-help cognitive behaviour therapy for working women with menopausal symptoms (MENOS@ Work). Maturitas 2016;92:186–92.

144. Norton S, Chilcot J, Hunter MS. Cognitive-behavior therapy for menopausal symptoms (hot flushes and night sweats): moderators and mediators of treatment effects. Menopause 2014;21(6):574–8.

145. Stefanopoulou E, Hunter MS. Telephone-guided self-help cognitive behavioural therapy for menopausal symptoms. Maturitas 2014;77(1):73–7.

146. Carpenter JS, Neal JG, Payne J, et al. Cognitive-behavioral intervention for hot flashes. Oncol Nurs Forum 2007;34(1):37.

147. Thomas A, Grandner M, Nowakowski S, et al. Where are the behavioral sleep medicine providers and where are they needed? a geographic assessment. Behav Sleep Med 2016;14(6):687–98.

Delivering Cognitive Behavioral Therapy for Insomnia in Military Personnel and Veterans

Monica R. Kelly, PhD[a], Ruth Robbins, PhD[b],
Jennifer L. Martin, PhD[a,c],*

KEYWORDS

- Cognitive-behavioral therapy for insomnia • Military • Veteran • Post-traumatic stress disorder
- Depression • Aging • Sleep apnea • Chronic pain

KEY POINTS

- Insomnia is frequently reported by active-duty military personnel and veterans.
- There is a bidirectional relationship between insomnia and mental or physical heath disorders that commonly occur in military populations.
- Cognitive-behavioral therapy for insomnia (CBT-I) is efficacious in improving sleep and functioning in military populations from active-duty service members to older veterans.
- Military personnel and veterans with complex presentations including post-traumatic stress disorder, depression, sleep apnea, and chronic pain benefit from CBT-I.
- Data evaluating CBT-I are limited in women service members and veterans, as well as individuals with substance use disorders, despite high prevalence and risk of sleep difficulties in these subgroups.

INTRODUCTION

Insomnia is one of the 2 most commonly diagnosed sleep disorders among military service members and veterans. Both the Department of Defense (DOD) and Veterans Administration (VA) have embraced cognitive-behavioral therapy for insomnia (CBT-I) as a valuable first-line approach to treatment, conducting large-scale provider training initiatives to meet the needs of individuals served by these 2 large health care systems.[1]

Insomnia disorder seldom occurs on its own in service members and veterans; rather, it is typically seen in the context of other physical and mental health conditions. It is also more common among women service members and veterans in comparison with men, although treatment studies with military populations have included a predominance of men (typically 80% to 90%) with some studies including exclusively men.[2,3] Results of randomized controlled trials and clinical implementation of CBT-I show that it retains its effectiveness when delivered to service

Disclosures: The authors have no potential conflicts of interest to disclose. This work was supported by the VA Greater Los Angeles Healthcare System, Geriatric Research, Education and Clinical Center, and NIH/NHLBI K24HL143055 (principal investigator: J.L. Martin).
a Geriatric Research, Education and Clinical Center, VA Greater Los Angeles Healthcare System, VA Sepulveda Ambulatory Care Center, 11E, 16111 Plummer Street, North Hills, CA 91343, USA; b VA Greater Los Angeles Healthcare System, Department of Psychology, VA Sepulveda Ambulatory Care Center, 16111 Plummer Street, North Hills, CA 91343, USA; c Department of Medicine, David Geffen School of Medicine, University of California, Los Angeles, 10833 Le Conte Ave, Los Angeles, CA 90095, USA
* Corresponding author. Geriatric Research, Education and Clinical Center, VA Greater Los Angeles Healthcare System, VA Sepulveda Ambulatory Care Center, 11E, 16111 Plummer Street, North Hills, CA 91343, USA
E-mail address: Jennifer.Martin@va.gov

members and veterans in "real-world" clinical practice, even in the context of comorbid conditions.[1,4]

MENTAL HEALTH COMORBIDITIES

In service members and veterans, insomnia disorder commonly co-occurs with mental health conditions, an association that has adverse consequences for functioning. Disrupted sleep is also a risk factor for mental health disorders, including post-traumatic stress disorder (PTSD) and depression. A recent study of active-duty Army personnel found that insomnia is highly comorbid with major depressive disorder (85%), generalized anxiety disorder (83%), and PTSD (70%).[5] The relationship between insomnia and mental health symptoms is bidirectional and chronic in nature. Insomnia symptoms before deployment are predictive of a greater risk for development of depression, anxiety, and PTSD,[6] and sleep difficulties are also core diagnostic criteria of PTSD and depression.[7] Younger veterans deployed during Operation Iraqi Freedom/Operation Enduring Freedom/Operation New Dawn (OEF/OIF/OND) with premorbid psychiatric disorders are more likely to suffer from insufficient and poor quality sleep compared to those without premorbid psychiatric conditions, further supporting a bidirectional relationship between sleep and psychiatric illness.[8]

Post-traumatic Stress Disorder

Insomnia is the most frequently endorsed symptom of PTSD in service members after deployment,[9] and evidence suggests CBT-I is highly effective in improving sleep and reducing trauma symptoms in veterans with PTSD. Nearly half of Vietnam-era veterans with combat-related PTSD endorse regular difficulties with sleep onset and fragmentation.[10] Furthermore, insomnia is the most commonly reported enduring symptom following PTSD treatment in active-duty service members[11] and in individuals exposed to trauma at night.[12] Insomnia is also a predictor of poor response to exposure therapy for PTSD.[13] These findings suggest that veterans meeting the criteria for insomnia disorder and PTSD may benefit from sleep-focused interventions in multiple ways.

Some sleep symptoms present differently for individuals with military-related PTSD, particularly symptoms of hyperarousal at night. Veterans with PTSD show greater night-to-night and person-to-person variability in sleep symptoms[14] and distinctive maladaptive cognitions such as fear of re-experiencing nocturnal traumatic events or losing the ability to maintain vigilance during sleep.[15] These hypervigilance-related features may be related to the context of the trauma (ie, sexual assault in bed, night-time combat), and manifest behaviorally through actions such as trying to avoid falling asleep, checking behaviors, and keeping weapons at the bedside. A theoretic model describing factors that predispose, precipitate, and perpetuate insomnia (the "3 P's" model of insomnia)[16] can be applied in the case of PTSD (**Table 1**). Using this conceptualization within insomnia treatment in PTSD, it may be helpful to highlight factors such as regularity in sleep scheduling, addressing unhelpful thoughts with cognitive therapy, and using coping strategies (eg, relaxation, grounding, distraction) for distress and arousal at night.

Table 1
"3 P's" model of insomnia and PTSD in military populations

Predisposing Factors	Precipitating Factors	Perpetuating Factors
Elevate risk for developing insomnia and PTSD	Trigger insomnia and PTSD	Maintain insomnia and PTSD
Family history of sleep or anxiety problems	Military trauma exposure (eg, combat, sexual or interpersonal assault)	Behaviors (eg, irregular sleep/wake schedule, hypervigilance—checking locks)
Early-life trauma exposure	Change in military status (eg, deployment, discharge)	Cognitions (eg, fears of vulnerability or nightmares leading to sleep avoidance, distress regarding daytime consequences of sleep loss)
Mental health symptoms (eg, high stress reactivity, anxiety, depression)	Social/interpersonal life stressors (eg, divorce, childbirth)	Maladaptive coping strategies (eg, napping, substance use including alcohol or caffeine)
Medical conditions (eg, apnea, pain)	Economic/occupational stressors (eg, job loss, shift work)	Environmental factors (eg, light, temperature)

CBT-I confers significant benefit for veterans with PTSD in terms of reducing insomnia severity across subjective sleep measures, improving general functioning, reducing nightmares, and reducing sleep-related fear.[17,18] Similar reductions in symptoms of insomnia severity have also been demonstrated for veterans with comorbid PTSD and insomnia in residential programs,[19] and when CBT-I is delivered via telehealth.[20] CBT-I is a robust therapy for individuals with co-occurring insomnia and PTSD even when delivered to patient populations that may not be able to easily access outpatient mental health services.

More than 70% of patients with PTSD have chronic nightmares,[21] and combining nightmare-focused treatments with CBT-I is supported by several studies. Imagery rehearsal therapy (IRT) and exposure, rescripting, and relaxation therapy (ERRT) have demonstrated positive results for veterans with PTSD and insomnia when combined with CBT-I.[22] Combining CBT-I with IRT improved subjective sleep, insomnia severity, nightmare frequency, and overall PTSD symptoms.[23,24] Sleep measured objectively by actigraphy also improved in one study.[25] Cognitive-behavioral social rhythm therapy uses techniques from social rhythm therapy, CBT-I, and IRT and is associated with improved sleep-related and PTSD-related symptoms.[24] Combining CBT-I with ERRT may also be beneficial for general sleep outcomes, nightmare frequency, and nightmare-related distress.[26] Addressing nightmares and insomnia together therefore has significant advantages.

Depression

Depression is a common mental health condition among military personnel and veterans with insomnia. Sleep difficulties are both prodromal to and diagnostic of depression,[27] and insomnia is a risk factor for suboptimal depression treatment response,[28] chronicity,[29] and relapse after treatment of depression.[30] Even following successful treatment of depression insomnia symptoms frequently remain, even among individuals considered in remission.[31] In military populations, depression is often comorbid with other mental health diagnoses such as PTSD,[32] further complicating the clinical picture.[33–35] In addition, in military personnel poor sleep is related to increased suicidality and history of suicide attempts[36] over and above other risk factors.[37]

Patients with comorbid insomnia and depression may present with symptoms that complicate CBT-I delivery. For example, depressed individuals may have low motivation and may find it more difficult to adhere to treatment recommendations.[38]

Similarly, depressed individuals may have difficulty with components of CBT-I that require them to get out of bed when not sleeping. Patients with comorbid depression may benefit from better understanding and addressing common symptoms of depression, such as low mood and anhedonia, which are not considered core insomnia symptoms but can interfere with treatment progress. Behavioral activation through working together with the patient to identify previously enjoyable or mastery-oriented activities could address depression-related difficulty rising at a prescribed time as well as using the bed as a coping strategy. Other modifications to CBT-I may be helpful, such as motivational interviewing to enhance adherence, early-morning exposure to bright light to improve mood and stabilize sleep, scheduled worry time to address rumination, and relaxation techniques. Collaborating with prescribing physicians with regard to pharmacotherapy for depression is also essential to ensure that sleep is not adversely affected by antidepressant therapy. Results of the VA's CBT-I dissemination program shows that CBT-I reduces depression severity and suicidal ideation in the context of routine clinical care, suggesting that CBT-I should be offered to individuals with comorbid depression and insomnia.[39]

Substance Use Disorders

Insomnia and substance use often co-occur, frequently in conjunction with other mental health difficulties. Veterans often report using substances such as alcohol and marijuana to cope with insomnia symptoms,[40,41] and insomnia symptoms predict alcohol relapse for military personnel and veterans.[42] Although mental health conditions are risk factors for substance use disorders (SUD), the relationship between depression or PTSD symptoms and alcohol use is mediated by insomnia severity among veterans, suggesting complex relationships among psychiatric conditions, substance use, and sleep.[43] Importantly, sleep symptoms may not remit after PTSD treatment in dual-diagnosis substance use residential treatment programs,[44] but there is evidence that CBT-I may reduce the risk of substance use relapse among individuals with a comorbid mental health condition. Although substances such as alcohol and cannabis may induce drowsiness or relaxation, sleep fragmentation is increased as substances are metabolized, and tolerance to sedation develops with continued use.[45] CBT-I in substance users may require multimodel interventions for co-occurring diagnoses because problematic alcohol use is associated with reduced treatment adherence,[46] and treatment of insomnia typically is not initiated until the recovery phase of SUD. CBT-I techniques are practical and effective interventions for sleep disturbance in individuals with a history of SUD. Although alcohol use relapse rates may not be reduced by CBT-I,[47,48] a pilot study of veterans with cannabis use disorder found that the CBT-I Coach mobile app was effective in reducing cannabis use and improving sleep.[49] Despite evidence for the interrelationship between sleep disturbance and substance use, studies investigating the effectiveness of CBT-I for military populations with problematic substance use patterns are limited.

MEDICAL ISSUES
Pain

There exists a bidirectional relationship between insomnia and chronic pain, suggesting that symptoms of both must be addressed to improve functioning. Among individuals with chronic pain, 50% to 70% report significantly disrupted sleep.[50] Chronic pain may cause patients to remain in lighter stages of sleep,[51] and interrupted sleep can, in turn, decrease pain thresholds.[52,53] Insomnia is a risk factor for chronic pain after acute injury,[54] and experimentally induced pain disrupts sleep.[55] In older veterans, poor sleep is associated with worse next-day subjective pain ratings.[56] Sleep difficulties are endorsed by 90% of Operation Iraqi Freedom/Operation Enduring Freedom (OIF/OEF) veterans who present with the "polytrauma clinical triad" of chronic pain, TBI, and PTSD.[57,58] PTSD-related hyperarousal can disrupt sleep[59,60] and lower pain thresholds[61] (**Fig. 1**). This underscores the complexity of sleep in relation to polytrauma and overall health.

Multiple factors complicate insomnia treatment in the context of chronic pain. Assessing medication use and working with prescribers is important because pain medications may lead to disruptions in sleep,[61,62] worsen sleep apnea,[63] and impair cognition.[50] Dysfunctional beliefs about the pain-sleep relationship, and behaviors such as extended time in bed for "rest," may be linked to poorly managed pain and contribute to insomnia symptoms. Providing psychoeducation about sleep and pain, making pain-specific behavioral recommendations (ie, separate "sleep" and "rest" locations), using cognitive therapy techniques to challenge unhelpful beliefs, using behavioral activation with activity pacing, and providing relaxation strategies may be helpful for chronic pain patients with insomnia.

There is a positive effect of CBT-I on sleep and mood outcomes in patients with chronic pain[64–66]; however, despite improvements in sleep, differences in pain ratings from preintervention to postintervention are not always achieved.[67] Among OIF/OEF veterans with polytrauma, modified CBT-I in combination with prazosin reduced headache intensity and frequency, reduced daytime sleepiness, and improved cognitive performance.[68] Overall, improvements from CBT-I in sleep indices for comorbid insomnia and pain suggest that CBT-I is a viable treatment option for patients with comorbid chronic pain and may improve their overall function.

Aging

Approximately one-half of older veterans endorse disturbed sleep,[69] and chronic, untreated sleep disturbances are associated with increased risk for negative physical,[70] psychological,[71] cognitive,[72–74] and social[75] outcomes. CBT-I is effective as a first-line treatment of insomnia in older adults,[76–78] and hypnotic medications are not recommended because of the risk for adverse effects.[79] The likelihood of taking sedative-hypnotic

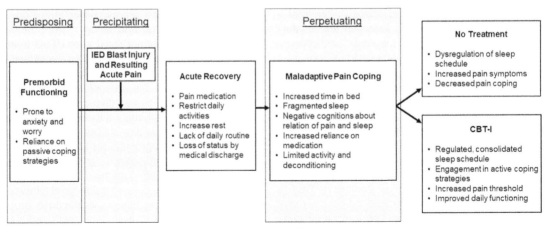

Fig. 1. Sleep and pain interact and affect implementation of insomnia treatment.

medications to treat sleep difficulties is higher in older adults, although they increase the risk for falls,[80,81] fractures,[82] strokes,[83] and mortality.[84] Studies of older veterans show benefit of CBT-I,[4,69] although older veterans underuse behavioral health services, posing unique challenges in delivering CBT-I to older veterans.[4,78,85]

Adaptations to CBT-I can be made to accommodate the physical and cognitive changes associated with advanced age.[86] Older adults may adopt unhelpful expectations regarding sleep and aging,[87] and psychoeducation is important to address these maladaptive thoughts. In addition, engagement in stimulating evening activities and eliminating activities that increase the risk of evening dozing are important tools in implementing CBT-I. To accommodate physical limitations and maintain safety from falls at night, modification to stimulus control instructions may be required. A recent study showed that CBT-I, delivered by trained non–mental health providers, produced significant improvements in sleep initiation and maintenance in older veterans and reported that benefits were sustained over a 12-month follow-up.[69] A second study explored benefits of an adapted version of CBT-I for older veterans in an Adult Day Health Care program and found benefits for this population for whom mild cognitive impairment, functional limitations, and limited social milieu are all commonplace.[86]

Sleep Apnea

Insomnia and obstructive sleep apnea (OSA) frequently co-occur[88] and contribute to impairments in functioning and quality of life, over and above either disorder in isolation.[89] Risk factors for OSA include obesity, use of central nervous system depressants (ie, opioids, alcohol), older age, male sex, and smoking.[90] Data from active-duty military personnel indicate increases in medical encounters for both insomnia and OSA.[91] More than 65% of active-duty personnel with PTSD have comorbid OSA,[92] and OSA is the most commonly diagnosed sleep disorder among VA users.[2] OSA is typically comorbid with medical conditions such as hypertension, cardiovascular diseases, and diabetes, and is associated with increased mortality[93,94] and psychiatric disorders including depression, anxiety, and PTSD.[90,95] Although the first-line treatment of OSA, positive airway pressure (PAP) therapy,[96] can improve sleep-related symptoms and health,[97] comorbid insomnia is associated with lower PAP adherence,[98] suggesting that CBT-I is an appropriate adjunctive therapy for OSA patients with insomnia.

Special treatment considerations or modifications may be needed to address compliance with PAP in veterans with comorbid OSA and insomnia. Early PAP use is predictive of long-term PAP adherence[99]; therefore, to encourage long-term PAP use, early intervention for insomnia is important. A Cochrane review reported that behavioral and educational interventions effectively improve PAP adherence,[100] and this can easily be woven into CBT-I treatments. In fact, interventions targeting veterans with coexisting OSA and insomnia have demonstrated positive sleep and PAP adherence outcomes.[101,102] Taken together, the literature provides support for using CBT-I in veterans with comorbid insomnia and OSA, and significant sleep-related benefits can be achieved. The available literature is currently limited in terms of studies assessing the role of CBT-I in OSA for active-duty populations, in which additional challenges to PAP use are present.

ACCESS TO CARE

Because insomnia is highly prevalent in the veteran population, and CBT-I has demonstrated effectiveness in patients with complex medical and mental health histories, a system-wide dissemination has been implemented by the VA and DOD.[1] The CBT-I dissemination program uses didactic and competency training components through lectures and telephone-based consultation about ongoing cases for mental health providers from a variety of disciplines. Outcomes demonstrate high success rates for provider competency[1] and self-efficacy,[103] in addition to large effects for improvement in insomnia symptoms for veterans.[4]

Despite these efforts, there are still barriers to engaging in CBT-I for military populations, such as the limited access to care and the stigma of mental health care. VA/DOD guidelines recommend CBT-I as a first-line treatment of insomnia disorder in PTSD[104]; however, veterans with insomnia and PTSD remain likely to receive sedative-hypnotic medications instead.[105] It may be the case that providers are unaware of CBT-I or the service may not be readily available (eg, limited to weekday sessions during standard work hours and larger, urban clinics). In addition to the provider training initiatives already described, alternative delivery modalities have been explored as a means of increasing access to CBT-I. There is evidence that small-group CBT-I is as effective as individual CBT-I for veterans.[106] Telehealth interventions for veterans in rural areas are also effective and may enable trained providers to more easily reach veterans living in remote areas.[20] Although Internet-based delivery may further increase access, available evidence suggests that it is inferior to face-to-face treatment for active-duty military personnel.[107]

Aside from systemic barriers to accessing CBT-I, there are also individual beliefs about mental health treatment, which are more prevalent in veterans who have been diagnosed with a mental health condition such as PTSD or depression, are younger, or identify as a racial/ethnic minority.[108] Nonetheless, one study of women veterans reported that patients actually prefer behavioral over pharmacologic insomnia treatment.[109] Connecting active-duty military personnel and veterans with CBT-I through primary care or non–mental health settings may be a means of reducing stigma and promoting engagement.

SUMMARY

Insomnia is commonly reported by military populations, especially those with comorbid mental and physical health conditions. Co-occurring conditions may result in an altered presentation of insomnia symptoms, and complicate the provision of CBT-I, requiring supplementary assessment or modifications to traditional CBT-I techniques. CBT-I has consistently demonstrated positive outcomes for active-duty military personnel and veterans, even in the context of significant comorbidities such as PTSD, depression, sleep apnea, and chronic pain. Despite its promise, studies of CBT-I in some military populations, including women, active-duty service members, and active-duty and veteran patients with SUD, remain lacking. Access to care remains a challenge, which is being addressed via provider training initiatives and exploration of alternative delivery modalities.

REFERENCES

1. Karlin BE, Trockel M, Taylor CB, et al. National dissemination of cognitive behavioral therapy for insomnia in veterans: therapist- and patient-level outcomes. J Consult Clin Psychol 2013;81(5): 912–7.
2. Alexander M, Ray MA, Hebert JR, et al. The national veteran sleep disorder study: descriptive epidemiology and secular trends, 2000-2010. Sleep 2016;39(7):1399–410.
3. Babson KA, Wong AC, Morabito D, et al. Insomnia symptoms among female veterans: prevalence, risk factors, and the impact on psychosocial functioning and health care utilization. J Clin Sleep Med 2018;14(6):931–9.
4. Karlin BE, Trockel M, Spira AP, et al. National evaluation of the effectiveness of cognitive behavioral therapy for insomnia among older versus younger veterans. Int J Geriatr Psychiatry 2015;30(3): 308–15.
5. Brownlow JA, Klingaman EA, Boland EM, et al. Psychiatric disorders moderate the relationship between insomnia and cognitive problems in military soldiers. J Affect Disord 2017;221:25–30.
6. Gehrman P, Seelig AD, Jacobson IG, et al. Predeployment sleep duration and insomnia symptoms as risk factors for new-onset mental health disorders following military deployment. Sleep 2013; 36(7):1009–18.
7. APA. Diagnostic and statistical manual of mental disorders: DSM-5. Arlington (VA): American Psychiatric Association; 2013.
8. Ulmer CS, Van Voorhees E, Germain AE, et al. A comparison of sleep difficulties among Iraq/Afghanistan theater veterans with and without mental health diagnoses. J Clin Sleep Med 2015; 11(9):995–1005.
9. McLay RN, Klam WP, Volkert SL. Insomnia is the most commonly reported symptom and predicts other symptoms of post-traumatic stress disorder in U.S. service members returning from military deployments. Mil Med 2010;175(10):759–62.
10. Neylan TC, Marmar CR, Metzler TJ, et al. Sleep disturbances in the Vietnam generation: findings from a nationally representative sample of male Vietnam veterans. Am J Psychiatry 1998;155(7):929–33.
11. Pruiksma KE, Taylor DJ, Wachen JS, et al. Residual sleep disturbances following PTSD treatment in active duty military personnel. Psychol Trauma 2016;8(6):697–701.
12. Zayfert C, DeViva JC. Residual insomnia following cognitive behavioral therapy for PTSD. J Trauma Stress 2004;17(1):69–73.
13. Lopez CM, Lancaster CL, Gros DF, et al. Residual sleep problems predict reduced response to prolonged exposure among veterans with PTSD. J Psychopathol Behav Assess 2017;39(4):755–63.
14. Straus LD, Drummond SP, Nappi CM, et al. Sleep variability in military-related PTSD: a comparison to primary insomnia and healthy controls. J Trauma Stress 2015;28(1):8–16.
15. Hull A, Holliday SB, Reinhard M, et al. The role of fear of loss of vigilance and reexperiencing in insomnia among veterans. Mil Behav Health 2016;4(4):373–82.
16. Spielman AGP. The varied nature of insomnia. In: Hauri PJ, editor. Case studies in insomnia. New York: Springer; 1991.
17. Talbot LS, Maguen S, Metzler TJ, et al. Cognitive behavioral therapy for insomnia in posttraumatic stress disorder: a randomized controlled trial. Sleep 2014;37(2):327–41.
18. Kanady JC, Talbot LS, Maguen S, et al. Cognitive behavioral therapy for insomnia reduces fear of

sleep in individuals with posttraumatic stress disorder. J Clin Sleep Med 2018;14(7):1193–203.

19. DeViva JC, McCarthy E, Bieu RK, et al. Group cognitive-behavioral therapy for insomnia delivered to veterans with posttraumatic stress disorder receiving residential treatment is associated with improvements in sleep independent of changes in posttraumatic stress disorder. Traumatology 2018. https://doi.org/10.1037/trm0000152.

20. Laurel Franklin C, Walton JL, Raines AM, et al. Pilot study comparing telephone to in-person delivery of cognitive-behavioural therapy for trauma-related insomnia for rural veterans. J Telemed Telecare 2018;24(9):629–35.

21. Leskin GA, Woodward SH, Young HE, et al. Effects of comorbid diagnoses on sleep disturbance in PTSD. J Psychiatr Res 2002;36(6):449–52.

22. Ho FY, Chan CS, Tang KN. Cognitive-behavioral therapy for sleep disturbances in treating posttraumatic stress disorder symptoms: a meta-analysis of randomized controlled trials. Clin Psychol Rev 2016;43:90–102.

23. Ulmer CS, Edinger JD, Calhoun PS. A multicomponent cognitive-behavioral intervention for sleep disturbance in veterans with PTSD: a pilot study. J Clin Sleep Med 2011;7(1):57–68.

24. Haynes PL, Kelly M, Warner L, et al. Cognitive behavioral social rhythm group therapy for veterans with posttraumatic stress disorder, depression, and sleep disturbance: results from an open trial. J Affect Disord 2016;192:234–43.

25. Margolies SO, Rybarczyk B, Vrana SR, et al. Efficacy of a cognitive-behavioral treatment for insomnia and nightmares in Afghanistan and Iraq veterans with PTSD. J Clin Psychol 2013;69(10):1026–42.

26. Swanson LM, Favorite TK, Horin E, et al. A combined group treatment for nightmares and insomnia in combat veterans: a pilot study. J Trauma Stress 2009;22(6):639–42.

27. Baglioni C, Battagliese G, Feige B, et al. Insomnia as a predictor of depression: a meta-analytic evaluation of longitudinal epidemiological studies. J Affect Disord 2011;135(1–3):10–9.

28. Troxel WM, Kupfer DJ, Reynolds CF 3rd, et al. Insomnia and objectively measured sleep disturbances predict treatment outcome in depressed patients treated with psychotherapy or psychotherapy-pharmacotherapy combinations. J Clin Psychiatry 2012;73(4):478–85.

29. Pigeon WR, Hegel M, Unutzer J, et al. Is insomnia a perpetuating factor for late-life depression in the IMPACT cohort? Sleep 2008;31(4):481–8.

30. Dombrovski AY, Mulsant BH, Houck PR, et al. Residual symptoms and recurrence during maintenance treatment of late-life depression. J Affect Disord 2007;103(1–3):77–82.

31. Carney CE, Segal ZV, Edinger JD, et al. A comparison of rates of residual insomnia symptoms following pharmacotherapy or cognitive-behavioral therapy for major depressive disorder. J Clin Psychiatry 2007;68(2):254–60.

32. Marmar CR, Schlenger W, Henn-Haase C, et al. Course of posttraumatic stress disorder 40 years after the Vietnam war: findings from the national Vietnam veterans longitudinal study. JAMA Psychiatry 2015;72(9):875–81.

33. Ramsawh HJ, Fullerton CS, Mash HB, et al. Risk for suicidal behaviors associated with PTSD, depression, and their comorbidity in the U.S. Army. J Affect Disord 2014;161:116–22.

34. Curry JF, Aubuchon-Endsley N, Brancu M, et al. Lifetime major depression and comorbid disorders among current-era women veterans. J Affect Disord 2014;152-154:434–40.

35. Magruder KM, Frueh BC, Knapp RG, et al. Prevalence of posttraumatic stress disorder in Veterans Affairs primary care clinics. Gen Hosp Psychiatry 2005;27(3):169–79.

36. Pigeon WR, Pinquart M, Conner K. Meta-analysis of sleep disturbance and suicidal thoughts and behaviors. J Clin Psychiatry 2012;73(9):e1160–7.

37. Ribeiro JD, Pease JL, Gutierrez PM, et al. Sleep problems outperform depression and hopelessness as cross-sectional and longitudinal predictors of suicidal ideation and behavior in young adults in the military. J Affect Disord 2012;136(3):743–50.

38. Trivedi MH, Lin EH, Katon WJ. Consensus recommendations for improving adherence, self-management, and outcomes in patients with depression. CNS Spectr 2007;12(8 Suppl 13):1–27.

39. Trockel M, Karlin BE, Taylor CB, et al. Effects of cognitive behavioral therapy for insomnia on suicidal ideation in veterans. Sleep 2015;38(2):259–65.

40. Cucciare MA, Darrow M, Weingardt KR. Characterizing binge drinking among U.S. military Veterans receiving a brief alcohol intervention. Addict Behav 2011;36(4):362–7.

41. Metrik J, Bassett SS, Aston ER, et al. Medicinal versus recreational cannabis use among returning veterans. Transl Issues Psychol Sci 2018;4(1):6–20.

42. Williams EC, Frasco MA, Jacobson IG, et al. Risk factors for relapse to problem drinking among current and former US military personnel: a prospective study of the Millennium Cohort. Drug Alcohol Depend 2015;148:93–101.

43. Miller MB, DiBello AM, Carey KB, et al. Insomnia severity as a mediator of the association between mental health symptoms and alcohol use in young

adult veterans. Drug Alcohol Depend 2017;177: 221–7.

44. Colvonen PJ, Ellison J, Haller M, et al. Examining insomnia and PTSD over time in veterans in residential treatment for substance use disorders and PTSD. Behav Sleep Med 2018;1–12. https://doi.org/10.1080/15402002.2018.1425869.

45. Garcia AN, Salloum IM. Polysomnographic sleep disturbances in nicotine, caffeine, alcohol, cocaine, opioid, and cannabis use: a focused review. Am J Addict 2015;24(7):590–8.

46. Magura S, Mateu PF, Rosenblum A, et al. Risk factors for medication non-adherence among psychiatric patients with substance misuse histories. Ment Health Subst Use 2014;7(4):381–90.

47. Currie SR, Clark S, Hodgins DC, et al. Randomized controlled trial of brief cognitive-behavioural interventions for insomnia in recovering alcoholics. Addiction 2004;99(9):1121–32.

48. Arnedt JT, Conroy DA, Armitage R, et al. Cognitive-behavioral therapy for insomnia in alcohol dependent patients: a randomized controlled pilot trial. Behav Res Ther 2011;49(4):227–33.

49. Babson KA, Ramo DE, Baldini L, et al. Mobile app-delivered cognitive behavioral therapy for insomnia: feasibility and initial efficacy among veterans with cannabis use disorders. JMIR Res Protoc 2015;4(3):e87.

50. Menefee LA, Cohen MJ, Anderson WR, et al. Sleep disturbance and nonmalignant chronic pain: a comprehensive review of the literature. Pain Med 2000;1(2):156–72.

51. Moldofsky H. Sleep influences on regional and diffuse pain syndromes associated with osteoarthritis. Semin Arthritis Rheum 1989;18(4 Suppl 2):18–21.

52. Moldofsky H, Lue FA, Smythe HA. Alpha EEG sleep and morning symptoms in rheumatoid arthritis. J Rheumatol 1983;10(3):373–9.

53. Older SA, Battafarano DF, Danning CL, et al. The effects of delta wave sleep interruption on pain thresholds and fibromyalgia-like symptoms in healthy subjects; correlations with insulin-like growth factor I. J Rheumatol 1998;25(6):1180–6.

54. Finan PH, Goodin BR, Smith MT. The association of sleep and pain: an update and a path forward. J Pain 2013;14(12):1539–52.

55. Sutton BC, Opp MR. Musculoskeletal sensitization and sleep: chronic muscle pain fragments sleep of mice without altering its duration. Sleep 2014; 37(3):505–13.

56. Dzierzewski JM, Williams JM, Roditi D, et al. Daily variations in objective nighttime sleep and subjective morning pain in older adults with insomnia: evidence of covariation over time. J Am Geriatr Soc 2010;58(5):925–30.

57. Lew HL, Otis JD, Tun C, et al. Prevalence of chronic pain, posttraumatic stress disorder, and persistent postconcussive symptoms in OIF/OEF veterans: polytrauma clinical triad. J Rehabil Res Dev 2009; 46(6):697–702.

58. Lew HL, Pogoda TK, Hsu PT, et al. Impact of the "polytrauma clinical triad" on sleep disturbance in a department of veterans affairs outpatient rehabilitation setting. Am J Phys Med Rehabil 2010;89(6): 437–45.

59. Kobayashi I, Boarts JM, Delahanty DL. Polysomnographically measured sleep abnormalities in PTSD: a meta-analytic review. Psychophysiology 2007; 44(4):660–9.

60. Yetkin S, Aydin H, Ozgen F. Polysomnography in patients with post-traumatic stress disorder. Psychiatry Clin Neurosci 2010;64(3):309–17.

61. Onen SH, Alloui A, Gross A, et al. The effects of total sleep deprivation, selective sleep interruption and sleep recovery on pain tolerance thresholds in healthy subjects. J Sleep Res 2001;10(1): 35–42.

62. Morasco BJ, O'Hearn D, Turk DC, et al. Associations between prescription opioid use and sleep impairment among veterans with chronic pain. Pain Med 2014;15(11):1902–10.

63. Molony RR, MacPeek DM, Schiffman PL, et al. Sleep, sleep apnea and the fibromyalgia syndrome. J Rheumatol 1986;13(4):797–800.

64. Currie SR, Wilson KG, Pontefract AJ, et al. Cognitive-behavioral treatment of insomnia secondary to chronic pain. J Consult Clin Psychol 2000; 68(3):407–16.

65. Edinger JD, Wohlgemuth WK, Krystal AD, et al. Behavioral insomnia therapy for fibromyalgia patients: a randomized clinical trial. Arch Intern Med 2005;165(21):2527–35.

66. Rybarczyk B, Stepanski E, Fogg L, et al. A placebo-controlled test of cognitive-behavioral therapy for comorbid insomnia in older adults. J Consult Clin Psychol 2005;73(6):1164–74.

67. Jungquist CR, O'Brien C, Matteson-Rusby S, et al. The efficacy of cognitive-behavioral therapy for insomnia in patients with chronic pain. Sleep Med 2010;11(3):302–9.

68. Ruff RL, Ruff SS, Wang XF. Improving sleep: initial headache treatment in OIF/OEF veterans with blast-induced mild traumatic brain injury. J Rehabil Res Dev 2009;46(9):1071–84.

69. Alessi C, Martin JL, Fiorentino L, et al. Cognitive behavioral therapy for insomnia in older veterans using nonclinician sleep coaches: randomized controlled trial. J Am Geriatr Soc 2016;64(9):1830–8.

70. Song Y, Dzierzewski JM, Fung CH, et al. Association between sleep and physical function in older veterans in an adult day healthcare program. J Am Geriatr Soc 2015;63(8):1622–7.

71. Jaussent I, Bouyer J, Ancelin ML, et al. Insomnia and daytime sleepiness are risk factors for

depressive symptoms in the elderly. Sleep 2011; 34(8):1103–10.

72. Hahn EA, Wang HX, Andel R, et al. A change in sleep pattern may predict Alzheimer disease. Am J Geriatr Psychiatry 2014;22(11):1262–71.

73. Yaffe K, Falvey CM, Hoang T. Connections between sleep and cognition in older adults. Lancet Neurol 2014;13(10):1017–28.

74. Yaffe K, Nettiksimmons J, Yesavage J, et al. Sleep quality and risk of dementia among older male veterans. Am J Geriatr Psychiatry 2015;23(6):651–4.

75. Spira AP, Kaufmann CN, Kasper JD, et al. Association between insomnia symptoms and functional status in U.S. older adults. J Gerontol B Psychol Sci Soc Sci 2014;69(Suppl 1):S35–41.

76. Bloom HG, Ahmed I, Alessi CA, et al. Evidence-based recommendations for the assessment and management of sleep disorders in older persons. J Am Geriatr Soc 2009;57(5):761–89.

77. Morgenthaler T, Kramer M, Alessi C, et al. Practice parameters for the psychological and behavioral treatment of insomnia: an update. An American Academy of Sleep Medicine report. Sleep 2006; 29(11):1415–9.

78. Irwin MR, Cole JC, Nicassio PM. Comparative meta-analysis of behavioral interventions for insomnia and their efficacy in middle-aged adults and in older adults 55+ years of age. Health Psychol 2006;25(1):3–14.

79. Bertisch SM, Herzig SJ, Winkelman JW, et al. National use of prescription medications for insomnia: NHANES 1999-2010. Sleep 2014;37(2):343–9.

80. Stone KL, Blackwell TL, Ancoli-Israel S, et al. Sleep disturbances and risk of falls in older community-dwelling men: the outcomes of sleep disorders in older men (MrOS sleep) study. J Am Geriatr Soc 2014;62(2):299–305.

81. Diem SJ, Ewing SK, Stone KL, et al. Use of non-benzodiazepine sedative hypnotics and risk of falls in older men. J Gerontol Geriatr Res 2014;3(3):158.

82. Bakken MS, Engeland A, Engesaeter LB, et al. Risk of hip fracture among older people using anxiolytic and hypnotic drugs: a nationwide prospective cohort study. Eur J Clin Pharmacol 2014;70(7): 873–80.

83. Wu MP, Lin HJ, Weng SF, et al. Insomnia subtypes and the subsequent risks of stroke: report from a nationally representative cohort. Stroke 2014; 45(5):1349–54.

84. Weich S, Pearce HL, Croft P, et al. Effect of anxiolytic and hypnotic drug prescriptions on mortality hazards: retrospective cohort study. BMJ 2014; 348:g1996.

85. Karlin BE, Duffy M, Gleaves DH. Patterns and predictors of mental health service use and mental illness among older and younger adults in the United States. Psychol Serv 2008;5(3):275–94.

86. Martin JL, Song Y, Hughes J, et al. A four-session sleep intervention program improves sleep for older adult day health care participants: results of a randomized controlled trial. Sleep 2017;40(8). https://doi.org/10.1093/sleep/zsx079.

87. Morin CM, Stone J, Trinkle D, et al. Dysfunctional beliefs and attitudes about sleep among older adults with and without insomnia complaints. Psychol Aging 1993;8(3):463–7.

88. Hein M, Lanquart JP, Loas G, et al. Prevalence and risk factors of moderate to severe obstructive sleep apnea syndrome in insomnia sufferers: a study on 1311 subjects. Respir Res 2017;18(1):135.

89. Sweetman AM, Lack LC, Catcheside PG, et al. Developing a successful treatment for co-morbid insomnia and sleep apnoea. Sleep Med Rev 2017;33:28–38.

90. Colvonen PJ, Masino T, Drummond SP, et al. Obstructive sleep apnea and posttraumatic stress disorder among OEF/OIF/OND veterans. J Clin Sleep Med 2015;11(5):513–8.

91. A Caldwell J, Knapik JJ, Lieberman HR. Trends and factors associated with insomnia and sleep apnea in all United States military service members from 2005 to 2014. J Sleep Res 2017;26(5):665–70.

92. Williams SG, Collen J, Orr N, et al. Sleep disorders in combat-related PTSD. Sleep Breath 2015;19(1): 175–82.

93. Punjabi NM, Caffo BS, Goodwin JL, et al. Sleep-disordered breathing and mortality: a prospective cohort study. PLoS Med 2009;6(8):e1000132.

94. Solomon SD, Davidson JR. Trauma: prevalence, impairment, service use, and cost. J Clin Psychiatry 1997;58(Suppl 9):5–11.

95. Sharafkhaneh A, Giray N, Richardson P, et al. Association of psychiatric disorders and sleep apnea in a large cohort. Sleep 2005;28(11):1405–11.

96. Qaseem A, Holty JE, Owens DK, et al. Management of obstructive sleep apnea in adults: a clinical practice guideline from the American College of Physicians. Ann Intern Med 2013;159(7):471–83.

97. Orr JE, Smales C, Alexander TH, et al. Treatment of OSA with CPAP is associated with improvement in PTSD symptoms among veterans. J Clin Sleep Med 2017;13(1):57–63.

98. Pieh C, Bach M, Popp R, et al. Insomnia symptoms influence CPAP compliance. Sleep Breath 2013; 17(1):99–104.

99. Budhiraja R, Parthasarathy S, Drake CL, et al. Early CPAP use identifies subsequent adherence to CPAP therapy. Sleep 2007;30(3):320–4.

100. Wozniak DR, Lasserson TJ, Smith I. Educational, supportive and behavioural interventions to improve usage of continuous positive airway pressure machines in adults with obstructive sleep apnoea. Cochrane Database Syst Rev 2014;(1): CD007736.

101. Alessi CA, Martin JL, Fung CH, et al. 0407 Randomized controlled trial of an integrated behavioral treatment in veterans with obstructive sleep apnea and coexisting insomnia. Sleep 2018;41(suppl_1): A155.

102. Fung CH, Martin JL, Josephson K, et al. Efficacy of cognitive behavioral therapy for insomnia in older adults with occult sleep-disordered breathing. Psychosom Med 2016;78(5):629–39.

103. Manber R, Trockel M, Batdorf W, et al. Lessons learned from the national dissemination of cognitive behavioral therapy for insomnia in the Veterans Health Administration: impact of training on therapists' self-efficacy and attitudes. Sleep Med Clin 2013;8(3):399–405.

104. VA/DoD. VA/DoD clinical practice guideline for management of post-traumatic stress. Washington, DC: Department of Veterans Affairs, Department of Defense; 2017.

105. Bramoweth AD, Renqvist JG, Hanusa BH, et al. Identifying the demographic and mental health factors that influence insomnia treatment recommendations within a veteran population. Behav Sleep Med 2017;1–12. https://doi.org/10.1080/15402002.2017. 1318752.

106. Koffel E, Farrell-Carnahan L. Feasibility and preliminary real-world promise of a manualized group-based cognitive behavioral therapy for insomnia protocol for veterans. Mil Med 2014; 179(5):521–8.

107. Taylor DJ, Peterson AL, Pruiksma KE, et al. Internet and in-person cognitive behavioral therapy for insomnia in military personnel: a randomized clinical trial. Sleep 2017;40(6). https://doi.org/10. 1093/sleep/zsx075.

108. Pietrzak RH, Johnson DC, Goldstein MB, et al. Perceived stigma and barriers to mental health care utilization among OEF-OIF veterans. Psychiatr Serv 2009;60(8):1118–22.

109. Culver NC, Song Y, Kate McGowan S, et al. Acceptability of medication and nonmedication treatment for insomnia among female veterans: effects of age, insomnia severity, and psychiatric symptoms. Clin Ther 2016;38(11): 2373–85.

A Meta-Analysis of Mindfulness-Based Therapies for Insomnia and Sleep Disturbance
Moving Towards Processes of Change

Joshua A. Rash, PhD[a], Victoria A.J. Kavanagh, BA[a],
Sheila N. Garland, PhD[a,b],*

KEYWORDS

• Insomnia • Sleep • Mindfulness • Meta-analysis • Mechanisms

KEY POINTS

- The Psychological Process Model of Sleep postulates that interventions such as mindfulness can influence sleep by altering psychological flexibility pertaining to sleep through process variables (eg, awareness, decentering, acceptance, defusion, values, readiness to change, and motivation).
- Mindfulness-based treatments are efficacious at reducing symptoms of insomnia and improving sleep quality among adults when compared with psychological placebos and waitlist control conditions.
- Mindfulness-based interventions for sleep are characterized by conceptual and methodological heterogeneity.
- Future research is needed that evaluates mediators and moderators of intervention effects in an attempt to identify the empirically supported processes of change linking mindfulness-based interventions and sleep outcomes.

INTRODUCTION

Once a term only familiar to Buddhists and experienced meditators, "mindfulness" has quickly been taken up as a goal to be attained by the mainstream and is being applied to all aspects of daily life,[1] including sleep. Some have argued that the popularity of mindfulness may also contribute to its downfall, resulting from inappropriate application and misinformation about the effectiveness of mindfulness-based therapies (MBTs) as a consequence of poor methodology and weak theoretic underpinnings.[2] Although the larger community of mindfulness researchers have sounded the alarm,[3,4] it is unknown whether this has been heard by researchers who are investigating the application of MBTs for sleep.

Mindfulness has been described as an umbrella term "used to characterize a large number of practices, processes, and characteristics, largely

Disclosure statement: The authors do not have any commercial or financial conflicts of interest.
Funding: Dr S.N. Garland is funded by a New Investigator Award from the Beatrice Hunter Cancer Research Institute.
[a] Department of Psychology, Faculty of Science, Memorial University of Newfoundland, 232 Elizabeth Avenue, St John's, Newfoundland A1B 3X9, Canada; [b] Division of Oncology, Faculty of Medicine, Memorial University of Newfoundland, 300 Prince Phillip Drive, St John's, Newfoundland A1B 3V6, Canada
* Corresponding author. Department of Psychology, Memorial University of Newfoundland, 232 Elizabeth Avenue, St John's, Newfoundland A1B 3X9, Canada.
E-mail address: sheila.garland@mun.ca

defined in relation to the capacities of attention, awareness, memory/retention, and acceptance/discernment."[2] The definition of mindfulness most often cited comes from the seminal work by Jon Kabat-Zinn who characterized mindfulness as paying attention, on purpose, in the present moment without judgment.[5] Although this definition may be the most commonly cited, there remains little consensus on what mindfulness is, the specific mechanisms of effect, and how to measure the construct.[6] This creates several problems for researchers who are interested in applying and/or modifying and testing an intervention in a particular population such as those with insomnia and/or poor sleep.

Herein, the authors present a unifying model that can be used to understand how mindful practices, processes, and characteristics might be relevant to the normal sleep process and how acceptance- and mindfulness-based interventions may be used to target the mechanisms that perpetuate insomnia. Further, they undertook a review of the literature and performed a meta-analysis of randomized controlled trials (RCTs) evaluating the effect of MBTs on sleep among adults with insomnia or sleep problems with the following objectives:

1. To describe the methodological quality of the available research. The authors were particularly interested in assessing the frequency that research reported modifications to the intervention to make it specific to sleep and whether investigators assessed whether the mindfulness training was associated with, in part or in whole, sleep outcomes.
2. To assess the immediate (ie, postintervention) and sustained (ie, at follow-up) effects of MBTs for insomnia and sleep disturbance compared with waitlist or attention/education controls. Given the limited number and the variability in the nature of active comparison interventions, the authors thought it premature to compare MBTs with active controls at this time.
3. To propose a series of recommendations to guide future research in this area.

The Relationship Between Mindfulness and Sleep: Toward a Psychological Process Model of Sleep

From a theoretic perspective, there are several plausible mechanisms through which MBTs might operate to improve insomnia and associated daytime impairment. An understanding of normal sleep and the development of chronic insomnia is important to elucidating these mechanisms.

Sleep is a naturally unfolding process that is governed by homeostatic and circadian regulation.[7] Under normal circumstances, sleep-related reduction in arousal occurs automatically and passively (ie, without attention, intention, or effort).[8] The sleep system can be thought of as a self-calibrating system that maintains a degree of flexibility and returns to a homeostatic set-point following acute perturbations (eg, acute stressors that increase physiologic and cognitive/emotional arousal).

There have been 9 models proposed to explain the development of chronic insomnia.[9] Insomnia is theorized to be a disorder characterized by somatic, cognitive, and cortical hyperarousal.[8,10,11] Evidence from autonomic, neuroendocrine, immunology, and neuroimaging studies have generally supported the notion that insomnia is characterized by a failure to dearouse before sleep.[11,12] According to the 3P,[13] 4P,[14] and neurocognitive models,[10] predisposing factors (eg, hyperreactivity, proclivity to ruminate) serve as a diathesis toward the development of chronic insomnia that interact with precipitating factors and trigger acute disturbance in sleep continuity (eg, life stressors, psychiatric illness). Chronic insomnia is believed to develop within the context of perpetuating factors that interfere with the plasticity and automaticity of sleep and prevent the process of nighttime dearousal at the behavioral (eg, maladaptive habits and safety behaviors, such as spending excessive time in bed), cognitive (eg, dysfunctional beliefs about sleep and its consequences), and emotional levels (eg, paired associations between the bed and worry or frustration).[15–18]

Factors that perpetuate insomnia can be categorized as sleep-interfering, sleep-interpreting, and meta-cognitive processes.[17,19] Sleep-interfering processes include arousal-producing processes that interfere with sleep. Sleep-interpreting processes include dysfunctional beliefs, expectations and attributions concerning sleep, and the causes and consequences of poor sleep.[17] Meta-cognitive processes refer to the way that people relate to their thoughts about sleep, including rigidity in sleep-related behaviors and beliefs, attachment to sleep-related needs and expectations, and absorption in solving the sleep problem.[19] In reality, these processes feed into one another and result in a vicious cycle. For example, compared with good sleepers, people with insomnia endorse unhelpful beliefs about (1) the negative consequences of insomnia; (2) fear of losing control over sleep; and (3) helplessness about the unpredictability of sleep.[16,20,21] They describe their thoughts as intrusive, uncontrollable, and negative.[22,23] Individuals who suffer from insomnia report devoting greater effort toward sleep,[24] rigidity in beliefs about sleep, and attachment toward sleep-related needs and expectations.[19,25] Perhaps unsurprisingly, relative to controls, individuals with insomnia report the use of a higher number of sleep-interfering processes, including worry, thought suppression, and rumination.[26–30]

MBTs may improve sleep by facilitating psychological flexibility, improving meta-cognitive processes that contribute to insomnia, and promoting sleep-related dearousal. Psychological flexibility refers to (1) conscious and open contact with thoughts and feelings; (2) an awareness of the available responses in any situation; and (3) changing or persisting in behavior when doing so serves one's goals and values.[31,32] Psychological flexibility contains a set of 6 interrelated subprocesses, including (1) acceptance—the ability to open up to unwanted experiences without struggle or avoidance; (2) cognitive defusion—the ability to notice thoughts as thoughts rather than becoming wrapped up in their meaning; (3) being present—open, nonjudgmental contact with the present; (4) self-as-observer—seeing oneself as more than a collection of thoughts and feelings; (5) values—understanding chosen qualities of purposive action; and (6) committed action—development of larger patterns of effective actions linked to chosen values.[31,32] A cross-sectional assessment of 159 adults with chronic pain (79% with clinical insomnia) reported associations between components of psychological flexibility and symptoms of insomnia in the expected directions (ie, an inverse association between psychological flexibility and symptoms of insomnia).[33] Adopting psychological flexibility as an underlying model, MBTs can be used to explicitly target sleep-interfering, sleep-interpreting, and meta-cognitive processes that maintain insomnia, including: (1) fostering a willingness to accept unpleasant experiences, thoughts, and beliefs pertaining to sleep and the possibility that safety behaviors (eg, excess time spent in bed) may contribute to the sleep problem

rather than the sleep solution; (2) facilitating psychological distance from entrenched beliefs about sleep (ie, cognitive defusion, decentering, or disengagement) by promoting present focused, nonjudgmental awareness of thoughts, physical sensations, and feelings. This state of equanimity can serve to reduce the struggle with feelings, entanglement with arousing thoughts, and reliance on ineffective meta-cognitive processes, such as thought suppression; and (3) promoting committed action to values to reduce the focus on perceived daytime impairment.[19,25,34]

The adoption of an overarching psychological process model of sleep (PPMS; **Fig. 1**) to the treatment of insomnia is only useful to the extent that the model generates testable hypotheses that enrich our understanding of the disorder and its treatment. When viewed from this perspective, MBTs are viewed as targeting the process variables (ie, awareness, decentering, acceptance, defusion, values, readiness to change, motivation) that affect psychological flexibility[35] and have indirect effects on insomnia through reduction of sleep-related arousal. As such, it is important to perform a critical evaluation of the processes of change between MBTs and outcomes following the treatment of insomnia in order to advance our understanding of precision treatments for insomnia. This approach aligns with transdiagnostic treatments.[36] Treatments that target transdiagnostic processes (eg, cognitive rigidity and regulation of emotion) that underpin a broad range of diagnostic presentations, including insomnia and psychopathology, may be particularly effective among individuals with insomnia and medical/psychiatric comorbidity because they address a broader range of symptomatology.[37,38] One notable observational single-cohort study evaluated the processes of change in sleep problems following the delivery of group acceptance and commitment therapy for 252 patients with chronic pain and concomitant sleep problems, many of whom experienced comorbid depression. Treatment occurred on 4 days per week over

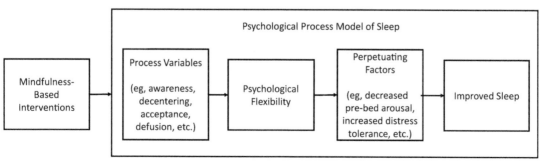

Fig. 1. How MBTs interact with the psychological process model of sleep.

4 weeks and included a prominent mindfulness component along with 2 hours of content on sleep that focused on sleep-related cognitions.[39] Significant improvement was observed for insomnia severity ($d = 0.45$), sleep interference ($d = 0.61$), sleep efficiency ($d = 0.32$), pain ($d = 0.72$), and symptoms of depression ($d = 1.03$), most of which were maintained at 9-month follow-up. Importantly, change was observed on measures of psychological flexibility (including acceptance and cognitive defusion), which were associated with sleep-related improvement.

The proposed psychological process model of sleep can be used to move past simply assessing whether MBTs can improve sleep and begin guiding future research questions on how MBTs exert their effect. It is also possible that applying such a mechanistic model will improve overall treatment efficacy, but this remains to be tested. While looking to the future, it is important to characterize the current literature pertaining to MBTs for insomnia and sleep disturbance to serve as a heuristic to inform the design of future trials. Two previous reviews and meta-analyses of the efficacy of MBTs specifically for sleep have been conducted, but these were characterized by limitations, including (1) the inclusion of study designs other than RCTs, (2) small or insufficient sample sizes, and (3) a failure to exclude studies where sleep was not the primary intervention target.[40,41] These limitations negatively affect the ability to draw firm conclusions. To appreciate the current state of the research applying MBTs to insomnia and sleep disturbance, the authors conducted a systematic review and meta-analysis of the literature with a focus on RCTs with sleep as the primary intervention target.

METHODS
Search Strategy

A thorough literature search was performed using 3 electronic databases—PubMed, Medline, and PsycInfo. Given the authors' interest in recent literature, search dates were restricted to January 01, 2010 to August 31, 2018. Searches were enhanced by scanning bibliographies of identified articles.

Search terms were constructed to include the combination of keywords and controlled vocabulary for 3 search themes, including mindfulness (eg, mindfulness or acceptance), sleep disturbance (eg, insomnia, sleep quality, and sleep disturbance), and RCTs. Terms within each theme were combined using the Boolean operator "OR." Themes were combined using the Boolean operator "AND."

Trial Selection

Articles were included if they met inclusion criteria for (1) trial design: reporting on an RCT; (2) trial population: adults older than 18 years with sleep disturbance, with clinically relevant levels of insomnia (as defined by the Diagnostic and Statistical Manual for Mental Disorders,[42] International Classification of Sleep Disorders[43] or the insomnia severity index [ISI])[21] or sleep disturbance (as defined by the Medical Outcomes Study Sleep Scale [MOS-SS],[44] Pittsburgh Sleep Quality Index [PSQI],[45] or sleep diary) at baseline; (3) delivery of an intervention where mindfulness/acceptance was a prominent component, including mindfulness-based stress reduction (MBSR), mindfulness-based cognitive therapy (MBCT), and acceptance and commitment therapy (ACT); and (4) outcome: measures of sleep (eg, sleep diary) or insomnia symptoms (eg, ISI) as a primary or secondary outcome. Only research published in English language journals were included.

Data Extraction

Details of each trial were extracted using a standardized extraction form. This form included the following information: author and year of published report, methods (eg, design of RCT, number of treatment arms, trial duration and follow-up, blinding, allocation concealment, method of randomization and attrition), participant characteristics (eg, sample size, age, sex distribution), control details, and outcomes. A separate table was used to record raw outcome data on symptoms of insomnia and sleep quality.

Quality Ratings

All trials were rated using a scale originally developed to assess the quality of psychological treatments for chronic pain.[46] The measure contains 2 subscales. The subscale measuring treatment quality evaluates stated rationale for treatment, manualization, therapist training, and patient engagement (scores range from 0–9 with higher scores reflecting greater rigor). The subscale measuring trial design and methods includes 8 items and evaluates inclusion/exclusion criteria, attrition, sample description, minimization of bias (randomization method, allocation bias, blinding of assessment, and equality of treatment expectations), selection of outcomes, length of follow-up, analyses, and choice of control (scores range from 0–26 with higher scores reflecting greater rigor). Scores on both subscales are summed to measure overall trial quality (scores range from 0–35). All trials were independently rated and consensus reached after initial comparison ratings.

Quantitative Data Synthesis

Procedures and formula for conducting a meta-analysis were based on recommendations by Lipsey and Wilson.[47] True effects estimates were computed as adjusted standardized mean differences (Hedge's g) using random effects models. Three steps were taken to calculate Hedge's g. First, the mean within-group difference was calculated as change from pretest to posttest within each trial. Second, prepost within-group standard deviations were pooled to calculate the standard deviation of change scores according to recommendations.[48] Finally, Hedge's g between the MBT and control groups was computed from the between-group change scores and associated standard deviation.

Pooling of effects and meta-analytic comparison was performed on trials that compared MBTs with inactive control conditions and psychological placebos (ie, attention/education controls). Meta-analysis was not performed on trials comparing an MBT with an active comparator because of the variability in active comparators. Separate meta-analyses were performed for effects at postintervention and follow-up. Fail-safe Ns were calculated to assess for publication bias using Orwin's formula.[49] The recommended criterion effect size of 0.20 was used.

Statistical analysis was performed using the random effects models performed with RevMan5.3 software (The Cochrane Collaboration, 2014). Heterogeneity was assessed using the I^2 index, chi-square, and tau^2 tests.[50] According to recommendations, substantial heterogeneity was assumed if I^2 exceeded 50%.[50]

Qualitative Analysis of Mindfulness and Sleep Components

The included papers were also evaluated based on the recommendations of Van Dam and colleagues[2] to improve reporting of mindfulness-based interventions. Extracted information included instructor details, experience and qualifications, mindfulness techniques used, home practice recommendations and tracking, use of supportive materials, monitoring of adverse events, and whether or not the participants had previous meditation experience. An additional column was added to specify whether the intervention was adapted or modified to include sleep-specific interventions or recommendations.

RESULTS
Summary of Included Trials

The search of the literature yielded 16 publications reporting on 13 trials conducted since 2010 that reported on 864 adults (542 women and 304 men). **Table 1** depicts the characteristics of included trials. Nine trials assessed the effect of MBTs on insomnia, with the remaining 4 investigating sleep disturbance more generally. Eight trials used an active control condition,[51–59] 3 an inactive control,[60–62] and 2 included both active and inactive control conditions.[63–66] Seven trials were conducted with adults with insomnia,[55,59,61,64,65] 2 of which were limited to older adults.[51,62] The remaining trials tested the intervention in cancer survivors,[53,57] veterans,[56,58] postmenopausal women,[52] and women with fibromyalgia.[60]

There was a great deal of heterogeneity between interventions tested. Three trials tested traditional MBSR interventions,[54,55,62] one trial used a modified MBSR protocol,[51] three trials tested combinations of MBTs with behavioral sleep approaches,[59,64,65] one combined mindfulness with relaxation training,[52] two used ACT practices tailored for sleep,[60,61] and three trials by the same group trained participants in focusing their awareness/attention without any formal meditation training.[56–58] The duration of the interventions ranged from a minimum of 2 weekly 1.5 hour sessions[58] to the maximally intensive 2.5 hour weekly classes for 8 weeks with daily assigned homework and a 6 hour silent retreat.[55,64] The overwhelming majority of the inventions tested were delivered in group format with only one delivered to individuals,[65] and one trial did not specify.[58]

Nine trials[51–53,56–59,61,65] included a measure of mindfulness but only 3 examined whether the measure of mindfulness was related to the sleep outcomes.[51,54,63] Three trials assessed whether self-reported minutes of meditation practice was associated with sleep outcomes.[55,59,64]

Trial Quality

Ratings of trial quality are presented in **Table 2**. Ratings for the reporting of treatment quality ranged from a low of 3 to a high of 9 (out of a possible 9). The areas of lowest quality were whether the treatment was manualized and whether formal checks on adherence to the manual by the therapists (ie, treatment fidelity) was conducted via direct observations, tape recording, or supervisory processes. The other most common area where trials were lacking was the inclusion of formal assessment of patient engagement, described as formal checks on homework or skills practice.

Table 1
Study details

RCTs that Assessed Effect of Mindfulness on Insomnia Symptoms with Active Control

First Author, Date	Sample/Sex Population	Intervention Details Follow-up Period	Control/Comparison Details	Sleep Outcome Mindfulness Outcome	Results	Relation Between Sleep & Mindfulness
Garcia et al,[52] 2018	30 Postmenopausal women w/insomnia (19 MRTI; 11 Control)	Group 8 wk (30 min/wk in class; up to 40 min/d at home) MRTI Follow-up: None	Group 8 wk Attention control general discussion in class (30 min) and crossword puzzles (up to 40 min)	Sleep: PSQI, ISI, polysomnography Mindfulness: MAAS	Relative to control, MRTI improved symptoms of insomnia and sleep quality. No differences between groups were observed for PSG variables. MAAS scores increased in the MRTI group only.	Not reported
Garland et al,[53] 2014 Garland et al,[54] 2015	111 (80 F; 31 M) patients with cancer w/insomnia (64 MBSR; 47 CBT-I)	Group 8 wk (90 min/wk) + 6 h silent retreat. MBSR Follow-up: 3 mo	Group 8 wk (90 min/wk) CBT-I	Sleep: actigraphy, DBAS, ISI, PSQI, sleep diary Mindfulness: FFMQ	MBSR was inferior to CBT-I immediately after treatment but not at 3 mo follow-up. As a single-group, MBSR resulted in improvement in symptoms of insomnia, sleep quality, and dysfunctional beliefs about sleep at 3 mo follow-up.	Both groups increased "acting with awareness" and "nonjudging." Increases in mindfulness were associated with decreases in DBAS scores. Nonjudging was associated with decreased insomnia severity.

Study	Sample	Intervention	Control/Design	Measures	Results	Correlation
Gross et al,[55] 2011	27 (22 F; 8 M) adults w/insomnia (18 MBSR; 9 pharmacotherapy)	Group 8 wk (2.5 h/wk) + 6 h silent retreat MBSR. Information on sleep hygiene Follow-up: 3 mo	3 mg of Eszopiclone (nightly for 8 wk) Pharmacotherapy information on sleep hygiene	Sleep: sleep diary, Actigraphy, ISI, PSQI, DBAS, SSES Mindfulness: none	MBSR used in conjunction with readings on sleep showed similar results to that of pharmacotherapy.	Significant correlation between reduction in dysfunctional sleep beliefs and meditation practice during intervention period.
Ong et al,[66] 2014; Ong et al,[64] 2018	54 (40 F; 14 M) adults w/insomnia (13 MBSR; 15 MBTI; 16SM)	Group 8 wk (2.5 h/wk) + 6 h silent retreat. MBSR or MBTI Follow-up: 3 mo, 6 mo	Individual 16 wk (8 wk SM, 8 wk BT) Delayed control	Sleep: GSES, BAS, HAS, FSS, ESS Mindfulness: none	MBSR and MBTI were superior to SM on all subjective and objective sleep measures but no significant differences found between MBSR and MBTI. MBTI was noninferior to BT for reducing sleep effort, dysfunctional sleep beliefs, and hyperarousal.	Significant correlation between more minutes of meditation and reduced dysfunctional sleep beliefs in MBTI group only.
Wong et al,[65] 2016 Lee et al,[63] 2018	64 (36 F; 21 M) adults w/insomnia (12 immediate MBT; 17 immediate CT; 14 delayed MBT; 14 delayed CT)	4 wk individual CBT-I followed by immediate MBT or CT Follow-up: 3 mo	4 wk individual CBT-I followed by 4 wk waiting then assignment to MBT or CT	Sleep: ISI, PSQI, APSQ, SAMI, DBAS, SRBQ, sleep diary, actigraphy Mindfulness: KIMS, NRI	After initial treatment with CBT-I, further treatment with MBT or CT produced further impairment, relative to WLC. No differences were observed between MBT and CT. MBT improved mindfulness skills (KIMS) and DBAS.	Baseline insomnia severity and sleep beliefs, but not mindfulness, predicted posttreatment insomnia severity.

(continued on next page)

Table 1
(continued)

First Author, Date	Sample/Sex Population	Intervention Details Follow-up Period	Control/Comparison Details	Sleep Outcome Mindfulness Outcome	Results	Relation Between Sleep & Mindfulness
Wong et al,[59] 2017	216 (169 F; 47 M) adults w/insomnia (111 MBCT-I; 105 PEEC)	Group 8 wk (2.5 h/wk) MBCT-I Follow-up: 5 mo, 8 mo	Group 8 wk (2.5 h/wk) PEEC	Sleep: ISI, sleep diary Mindfulness: FFMQ	The MBCT-I group was significantly better than the PEEC group posttreatment but not at 3 and 6 mo follow-ups. The MBCT-I group had greater reductions in WASO posttreatment and 3 mo. No other significant differences between PEEC and MBCT-I were observed. No change demonstrated on the FFMQ.	No differences in insomnia was seen in those who practiced their mediations 3x/week and those who did not.

RCTs that Assessed Effect of Mindfulness on Sleep Disturbance with Active Control

Black et al,[51] 2015	49 (33 F; 16 M) older adults w/sleep disturbance (24 MAPs; 25 SHE)	Group 6 wk (2 h/wk) MAPS Follow-up: none	Group 6 wk (2 h/wk) SHE	Sleep: FSI, PSQI, AIS Mindfulness: FFMQ	Relative to SHE, MAPS improved sleep quality, insomnia symptoms, depressed mood, and fatigue.	Mindfulness increased in MAPS but not SHE group. In the MAPS group, increased nonreactivity was associated with reductions in sleep disturbance and insomnia symptoms.

Study	Participants	Intervention	Control	Measures	Results	
Nakamura et al,[58] 2011	58 (3 F; 55 M) US veterans with sleep disturbance (33 MBB; 25 SHE)	2 wk (1.5 h/wk) MBB Follow-up: none	2 wk (1 h/wk) SED and monitoring using sleep diary	Sleep: MOS-SS Mindfulness: FFMQ	Larger reductions in sleep disturbance and greater increases in mind fulness were reported in the MBB group compared with the SED group at follow-up.	Not reported
Nakamura et al,[57] 2013	57 (43 F; 14 M) Cancer survivors with sleep disturbance (19 MBB; 20 MM; 18 SHE)	Group 3 wk (2 h/wk) MBB or MM Follow-up: none	Group 3 wk (2 h/wk) SED	Sleep: MOS-SS Mindfulness: FFMQ	Sleep disturbance improved in both the MBB and MM groups compared with SED, and mindfulness increased in MBB but not the MM group relative to SHE.	Not reported
Nakamura et al,[56] 2017	60 (6 F; 54 M) Gulf war veterans with sleep disturbance (33 MBB; 27 SHE)	Group 3 wk (2 h/wk) MBB Follow-up: 3 mo	Group 3 wk (2 h/wk) SED	Sleep: MOS-SS, MFI Mindfulness: FFMQ	No overall differences in sleep disturbance between MBB and SED immediately after treatment but MBB reported greater improvement than SED at follow-up. No reliable change in mindfulness.	Not reported
RCTs that Assessed Effect of Mindfulness on Insomnia Symptoms with Inactive Control						
Amutio et al,[60] 2018	39 female adults w/ fibromyalgia w/ insomnia (20 FM; 19 control)	Group 7 wk (2 h/wk) FM Follow-up: 3 mo	WLC	Sleep: AIS, PSQI, ESS, SII Mindfulness: none	The FM group improved sleep quality, sleepiness, sleep impairment, and subjective insomnia from pretest to posttest. These improvements continued during follow-up.	Not reported

(continued on next page)

Table 1
(continued)

First Author, Date	Sample/Sex Population	Intervention Details Follow-up Period	Control/Comparison Details	Sleep Outcome Mindfulness Outcome	Results	Relation Between Sleep & Mindfulness
deok Baik,[61] 2015	25 (16 F; 9 M) adults w/insomnia (14 ACT; 11 Control)	Group 2 wk (3–4 h/wk) ACT Follow-up: none	WLC, monitored sleep	Sleep: ISI, PSAS, sleep diary Mindfulness: AAQ-II, EQ	There was no effect of group on insomnia symptoms, presleep arousal, or sleep diary variables. Time effects were seen for both groups on measures of acceptance and mindfulness	Not reported
Zhang, 2015	60 (25 F; 35 M) older adults w/insomnia (30 MBSR; 30 control)	Group 8 wk (2 h/wk) + 2 h silent retreat MBSR Follow-up: none	WLC	Sleep: PSQI Mindfulness: none	Relative to WLC, MBSR improved PSQI total score and daytime dysfunction, but no other PSQI subscales	Not reported

Abbreviations: AAQ-II, acceptance and action questionnaire II; ACT, acceptance and commitment therapy; AIS, athens insomnia scale; APSQ, anxiety and preoccupation with sleep questionnaire; BAS, beliefs and attitudes about sleep scale; BT, behavioral therapy; CBT-I, cognitive behavior therapy for insomnia; CT, cognitive therapy; DBAS, dysfunctional beliefs and attitudes about sleep scale; EQ, experiences questionnaire; ESS, epworth sleepiness scale; F, female; FF-MQ, five facet mindfulness questionnaire; FM, flow meditation; FSI, fatigue symptom inventory; FSS, fatigue severity scale; GSES, glasgow sleep effort scale; HAS, hyper arousal scale; ISI, insomnia severity index; ISQ, insomnia symptom questionnaire; KIMS, Kentucky inventory of mindfulness skills; M, male; MAAS, mindfulness awareness attention scale; MAPS, mindfulness awareness practices intervention; MBB, mind body bridging; MBCT, mindfulness based cognitive therapy; MBCT-I, mindfulness-based cognitive therapy for insomnia; MBTI, mindfulness based therapy for insomnia; MFI, multidimensional fatigue inventory; MM, mindfulness meditation; MRTI, mindfulness and relaxation training for insomnia; NRI, nonreactivity to inner-experience; PEEC, psycho education with exercise control; PSAS, presleep arousal scale; PSD, Pittsburgh sleep diary; PSG, polysomnography; SAMI, sleep associative monitoring index; SED, sleep education; SHE, sleep hygiene education; SII, sleep impairment index; SM, self-monitoring; SRBQ, sleep-related behavior questionnaire; SSES, sleep self-efficacy scale; TCQIR, thought control.

Table 2
Study quality rating scale

Quality Rating	Amutio et al,[60] 2018	deok Baik,[61] 2015	Black, 2015	Garcia et al,[52] 2018	Garland et al,[53] 2014	Gross et al,[55] 2011	Nakamura et al,[58] 2011	Nakamura et al,[57] 2013	Nakamura et al,[56] 2017
Treatment Quality									
Treatment content 0,2	1	2	2	1	2	2	1	2	2
Treatment duration 0,1	1	1	1	1	1	1	1	1	1
Manualization 0,2	0	2	2	2	2	2	0	0	0
Manual adherence 0,1	0	1	0	0	0	0	0	0	0
Therapist training 0,2	1	2	2	0	2	2	1	1	1
Patient engagement 0,1	1	1	0	1	0	1	0	0	0
Overall treatment quality	4	9	7	5	7	8	3	4	4
Quality of Design and Methods									
Sample criteria 0,1	1	1	1	1	1	1	1	1	1
Evidence criteria met 0,1	1	1	1	1	1	1	1	1	1
Attrition 0,2	0	0	2	1	2	1	1	2	2
Rates of attrition 0,1	1	0	1	1	1	1	1	1	1
Sample characteristics 0,1	1	1	1	1	1	1	0	1	1
Group equivalence 0,1	1	1	1	1	1	0	1	0	1
Randomization 0,2	0	1	2	0	1	2	1	1	1
Allocation bias 0,1	1	0	1	0	1	1	0	0	0
Measurement bias 0,1	0	0	1	0	0	0	0	0	0
Treatment expectations 0,1	0	0	0	0	0	0	0	0	1
Justification of outcomes 0,2	2	2	2	2	2	2	2	2	2
Validity of outcomes 0,2	2	2	2	2	2	2	2	2	2
Reliability 0,2	2	2	2	2	2	2	2	2	2
Follow-up 0,1	0	0	0	0	0	0	0	0	0
Power calculation 0,1	0	0	1	0	1	0	0	0	1
Sample size 0,1	0	0	1	1	1	0	0	0	0
Data analysis 0,1	1	1	1	1	1	1	1	1	1
Statistics reporting 0,1	1	1	1	1	1	1	1	1	1

(continued on next page)

Table 2
(continued)

Quality Rating	Amutio et al,[60] 2018	deok Baik,[61] 2015	Black, 2015	Garcia et al,[52] 2018	Garland et al,[53] 2014	Gross et al,[55] 2011	Nakamura et al,[58] 2011	Nakamura et al,[57] 2013	Nakamura et al,[56] 2017
Intent to treat analysis 0,1	1	0	1	1	1	0	1	1	1
Control group 0,2	0	0	2	1	2	1	0	2	1
Overall design quality	14	13	24	17	22	17	15	18	20
Quality score	18	22	31	22	29	25	18	22	24

Quality Rating	Ong et al,[64] 2018	Wong et al,[65] 2016	Wong et al,[59] 2017	Zhang et al,[62] 2015
Treatment Quality				
Treatment content 0,2	2	2	2	1
Treatment duration 0,1	1	1	1	1
Manualization 0,2	1	2	1	2
Manual adherence 0,1	1	0	1	0
Therapist training 0,2	2	2	2	1
Patient engagement 0,1	1	0	1	0
Overall treatment quality	8	7	8	5
Quality of Design and Methods				
Sample criteria 0,1	1	1	1	1
Evidence criteria met 0,1	1	0	1	1
Attrition 0,2	2	1	2	1
Rates of attrition 0,1	1	1	1	1
Sample characteristics 0,1	1	0	1	1
Group equivalence 0,1	1	0	1	1
Randomization 0,2	2	1	2	1
Allocation bias 0,1	1	0	1	0
Measurement bias 0,1	0	0	1	0
Treatment expectations 0,1	1	0	0	0
Justification of outcomes 0,2	2	2	2	2
Validity of outcomes 0,2	2	2	2	2

Reliability 0,2	2	2	2	2
Follow-up 0,1	1	0	1	0
Power calculation 0,1	1	0	1	1
Sample size 0,1	0	0	1	1
Data analysis 0,1	1	0	1	1
Statistics reporting 0,1	1	1	1	1
Intent to treat analysis 0,1	1	1	1	1
Control group 0,2	2	2	2	0
Overall design quality	24	14	25	18
Quality score	32	21	33	23

Reporting of trial design and methods was also quite variable with a low of 13 to a high of 24 (out of a possible 26). Areas that trials were largely lacking were related to improper randomization and blinding procedures (the use of an independent person to create the allocation sequence or the use of sequentially numbered opaque sealed envelopes and using a third party who is blind to the patient's trial group for the collection of trial data), lack of a priori power calculations, and insufficient duration of follow-up (<6 months). Only 2 of the trials[56,64] included a measurement of participant treatment expectations, which is arguably a critical component of evaluations of behavioral trials.

The overall rating of trial quality was 24.62 across the 13 trials included. The original scale[46] did not include published cut-offs for overall quality; however, average scores for excellent, average, and poor trials across the validation sample were 22.70, 18.71, and 12.10, respectively. Thus, included trials would be considered excellent in trial quality when compared with RCTs of psychological interventions for adults with chronic pain. Combined, only 4 trials[51,53,59,64] had a total quality rating score in the top quarter (>26/35).

Meta-Analysis

Symptoms of insomnia

Six trials (n = 228; 76% women) reported on symptoms of insomnia, 5 using the Insomnia Severity Index and 1 using the Athens Insomnia Scale, and provided sufficient data for the computation of unbiased effect sizes[51,52,60,61,64,65] (**Fig. 2**). Meta-analysis of 3 trials with waitlist controls[60,61,65] indicated a main effect (g = 0.67, 95% confidence interval [CI] = 0.30–1.05, Z = 3.54,

$P<.01$) of MBTs for insomnia (n = 60) relative to waitlist controls (n = 58) at postintervention, with no heterogeneity across trials (I^2 = 0%, $\chi^2(2)$ = 0.15, P = .93). Meta-analysis of 3 trials with attention/education controls[51,52,64] indicated a main effect (g = 2.33, 95% CI = 0.37–4.29, z = 2.33, P = .02) of MBTs on insomnia (n = 58) relative to attention/education controls (n = 52) at postintervention, with significant heterogeneity across effects (I^2 = 93%, $\chi^2(2)$ = 27.64, P<.01).

Three trials reported on the effect of MBTs on symptoms of insomnia at 3-month follow-up[60,65,66] (**Fig. 3**). The effects of MBTs (n = 65) on symptoms of insomnia endured at 3-month follow-up (g = 1.06, 95% CI = 0.48–1.64) when compared with control (n = 49). It should be noted that this comparison is somewhat biased given that 2 trials[65,66] did not assess the control group at 3-month follow-up (ie, change in symptoms of insomnia due to MBT from baseline to 3-month follow-up was compared with change in control group from baseline to postintervention).

Sleep quality

Eight trials (n = 407; 52% women) reported on sleep quality, 5 using the PSQI and 3 using the MOS-SS SPI-II, and provided sufficient data for the computation of unbiased effect sizes[51,52,56–58,60,62,65] Meta-analysis of 3 trials[60,62,65] indicated a main effect (g = 1.17, 95% CI = 0.83–1.52, Z = 6.66, P<.01) of MBTs on sleep quality (n = 76) relative to waitlist control (n = 77) at postintervention, with no heterogeneity across trials (I^2 = 0%, $\chi^2(2)$ = 0.30, P = .86; **Fig. 4**). Meta-analysis of 5 trials[51,52,56–58] indicated a main effect (g = 1.10, 95% CI = 0.45–1.75, z = 3.31, P<.01) of MBTs on sleep quality

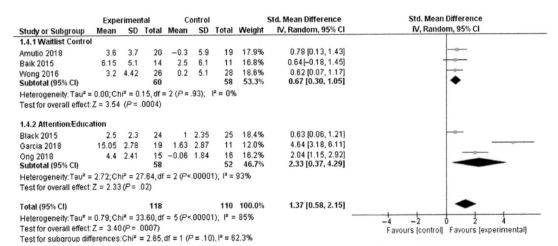

Fig. 2. Forest plot depicting the effect of MBTs on change in symptoms of insomnia from pretest to posttest. Separate forest plots are presented for waitlist and attention/education control conditions.

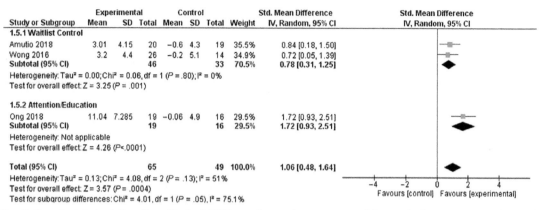

Study or Subgroup	Experimental			Control			Weight	Std. Mean Difference IV, Random, 95% CI	Std. Mean Difference IV, Random, 95% CI
	Mean	SD	Total	Mean	SD	Total			
1.5.1 Waitlist Control									
Amutio 2018	3.01	4.15	20	−0.6	4.3	19	35.5%	0.84 [0.18, 1.50]	
Wong 2016	3.2	4.4	26	−0.2	5.1	14	34.9%	0.72 [0.05, 1.39]	
Subtotal (95% CI)			46			33	70.5%	0.78 [0.31, 1.25]	

Heterogeneity: Tau² = 0.00; Chi² = 0.06, df = 1 (P = .80); I² = 0%
Test for overall effect: Z = 3.25 (P = .001)

1.5.2 Attention/Education									
Ong 2018	11.04	7.285	19	−0.06	4.9	16	29.5%	1.72 [0.93, 2.51]	
Subtotal (95% CI)			19			16	29.5%	1.72 [0.93, 2.51]	

Heterogeneity: Not applicable
Test for overall effect: Z = 4.26 (P<.0001)

| Total (95% CI) | | | 65 | | | 49 | 100.0% | 1.06 [0.48, 1.64] | |

Heterogeneity: Tau² = 0.13; Chi² = 4.08, df = 2 (P = .13); I² = 51%
Test for overall effect: Z = 3.57 (P = .0004)
Test for subgroup differences: Chi² = 4.01, df = 1 (P = .05), I² = 75.1%

Favours [control]   Favours [experimental]

Fig. 3. Forest plot depicting the effect of MBTs on change in symptoms of insomnia from pretest to 3-month follow-up. Separate forest plots are presented for waitlist and attention/education control conditions.

(n = 148) relative to attention/education controls (n = 106) at postintervention, with heterogeneity across trials (I^2 = 81%, $\chi^2(4)$ = 21.48, P<.01; see **Fig. 4**). A sensitivity test removing the article by Garcia and colleagues[52] diminished variability to 3% but did not change the overall effect.

Three trials reported on the effect of MBTs on sleep quality at 3-month follow-up,[56,60,65] and one trial at 2-month follow-up.[57] The effect of MBTs on sleep quality endured at follow-up (g = 0.81, 95% CI = 0.35–1.27, z = 3.43, P<.01) when pooled across inactive controls and psychological placebos (**Fig. 5**). It is important to note that one trial did not assess the control group at 3-month follow-up.[65]

Mindfulness Intervention Details and Sleep-Specific Components

Table 3 depicts the mindfulness intervention design features. The reporting of information

related to instructor experience, mindfulness training, and clinical qualifications was highly variable and sometimes vague. Only 6 trials[52,55,56,58,61,65] reported specific instructions to practice mindfulness skills in bed or during the middle of the night if awake. When stated, home practice recommendations ranged from 10 to 45 minutes per day. A little more than half of the trials (n = 7)[51,52,55,59–61,64] reported using logs to track meditation practice, whereas only 3 trials tracked adverse events.[51,59,66] Only 4 trials reported whether previous/current meditation experience was an inclusion criteria.[53,57,60,62]

Discussion

A systematic review of the literature for studies that reported on an MBT for the treatment of insomnia or sleep disturbance in adults yielded 13 trials published since 2010. Trials reported on diverse populations (eg, veterans, cancer

Study or Subgroup	Experimental			Control			Weight	Std. Mean Difference IV, Random, 95% CI	Std. Mean Difference IV, Random, 95% CI
	Mean	SD	Total	Mean	SD	Total			
1.3.1 Waitlist Control									
Amutio 2018	3.9	4.05	20	−0.7	3.2	19	11.9%	1.23 [0.54, 1.92]	
Wong 2016	2.6	3.91	26	−2.6	4.15	28	13.1%	1.27 [0.68, 1.86]	
Zhang 2016	3.33	2.95	30	−0.2	3.6	30	13.7%	1.06 [0.52, 1.60]	
Subtotal (95% CI)			76			77	38.7%	1.17 [0.83, 1.52]	

Heterogeneity: Tau² = 0.00; Chi² = 0.30, df = 2 (P = .86); I² = 0%
Test for overall effect: Z = 6.66 (P<.00001)

1.3.2 Attention/Education									
Black 2015	2.8	1.8	24	1.1	1.9	25	13.1%	0.90 [0.31, 1.49]	
Garcia 2018	8.21	1.7	19	2.18	1.84	11	7.1%	3.35 [2.18, 4.52]	
Nakamura 2011	27.36	16.05	33	12.92	20.4	25	13.7%	0.79 [0.25, 1.33]	
Nakamura 2013	22.71	15.39	39	7.72	17.26	18	13.2%	0.92 [0.34, 1.51]	
Nakamura 2017	19.5	18.75	33	13.5	16.56	27	14.1%	0.33 [−0.18, 0.84]	
Subtotal (95% CI)			148			106	61.3%	1.10 [0.45, 1.75]	

Heterogeneity: Tau² = 0.43; Chi² = 21.48, df = 4 (P = .0003); I² = 81%
Test for overall effect: Z = 3.31 (P = .0009)

| Total (95% CI) | | | 224 | | | 183 | 100.0% | 1.09 [0.69, 1.50] | |

Heterogeneity: Tau² = 0.23; Chi² = 23.87, df = 7 (P = .001); I² = 71%
Test for overall effect: Z = 5.33 (P<.00001)
Test for subgroup differences: Chi² = 0.04, df = 1 (P = .84), I² = 0%

Favours [control]   Favours [experimental]

Fig. 4. Forest plot depicting the effect of MBTs on change in sleep quality from pretest to posttest. Separate forest plots are presented for waitlist and attention/education control conditions.

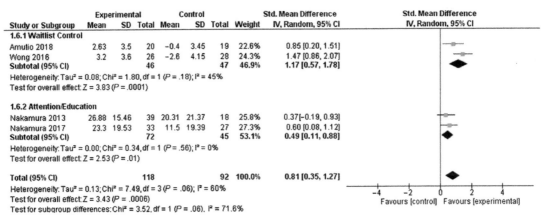

Fig. 5. Forest plot depicting the effect of MBTs on change in sleep quality from pretest to 3-month follow-up. Separate forest plots are presented for waitlist and attention/education control conditions.

survivors, individuals with fibromyalgia, and post-menopausal women) and used diverse MBTs (eg, MBSR, mindful bridging, MBCT, MBTI, ACT). Average trial quality was excellent, although substantial heterogeneity was observed between trials. Although the authors were unable to assess the effect of MBTs compared with other active treatments (such as cognitive behavior therapy for insomnia), the results of their meta-analysis indicated that MBTs are significantly more effective for reducing insomnia severity compared with attention/education and waitlist controls. The strength of this conclusion is limited by the significant heterogeneity among included trials. It can be concluded with stronger evidence that MBTs are significantly better than waitlist control groups and that the effects seem to be durable at 3 months postintervention. A similar pattern of results was observed for overall sleep quality.

This article represents an effort to present a unifying and testable theory for how mindfulness can be applied to the treatment of insomnia and sleep problems. MBTs are complimentary to behavioral and cognitive-behavioral approaches to treatment and can be used to augment existing treatments.[66,67] If MBTs operate at the level of psychological flexibility then they may exert their greatest effects on insomnia by facilitating patient adherence with challenging behavioral sleep interventions (eg, sleep restriction and stimulus control) while promoting mindful and nonjudgmental awareness of experience.[68] With this in mind, it will be important to progress from evaluating whether MBTs are effective for the treatment of insomnia and other sleep complaints to more refined questions as follows:

1. Are MBTs more effective when they are specifically tailored to sleep? Data pertaining to this question will inform whether mindfulness operates at the level of global psychological flexibility or psychological flexibility pertaining to solving the problem of perceived poor sleep.
2. Are MBTs an effective stand-alone treatment for insomnia? If so, does the addition of behavioral treatments for sleep significantly improve outcomes when added to MBTs.
3. What are the putative mechanisms (ie, processes of change) through which MBTs operate to improve sleep among individuals with insomnia or sleep disturbance?
4. For which individuals are MBTs most likely to be effective? For example, research evaluating MBTs for insomnia has focused on women (65% of the overall sample reviewed) and it is still unclear whether the effectiveness of MBTs for insomnia vary by patient sex.

Recommendation #1: Thoroughly Describe the Theory Justifying Why the Mindfulness-Based Therapy Being Tested Is Appropriate for the Treatment of Insomnia or Sleep Disturbance

It behooves researchers to provide more detailed justification for why the MBT is being proposed as a treatment for insomnia and/or poor sleep in their population of choice. The PPMS presents several testable hypotheses related to the theorized processes of change that can guide future research in this area.

Recommendation #2: Describe Whether the Mindfulness-Based Therapy Has Been Modified to Specifically Target the Proposed Mechanisms of Change and Solidify These in Manuals that Can Be Adopted by Others

Manualization is an important precursor to knowledge dissemination because it allows others to

Table 3
Mindfulness intervention design features

First Author, Year	Instructor Information				Intervention Details					Participant Information
	Instruction Experience	Mindfulness Training	Clinical Qualifications	Mindfulness Details	Specific Sleep Instructions	Meditation Practice/Log	Types of Materials	Monitoring of Adverse Events		Prior Experience with Meditation
Amutio et al,[60] 2018	Referred to as extensive	Referred to as extensive	Not reported	Formal meditation: body scan, breath awareness Acceptance and Commitment Therapy exercises and Zen meditation metaphors	Not reported	Home practice: 10 min/d of body scan, 30 min/d of full-body awareness breathing Log: daily record of level of engagement with at-home practices	Not reported	Not reported		Excluded if currently undergoing any mindfulness training
deok Baik,[61] 2015	Two previous training sessions	Not reported	Psychology graduate students	Formal meditation: sitting, metta, and tonglen meditation Awareness of body sensations, breathing, labeling thoughts, acceptance, commitment, and cognitive defusion	Tailoring of ACT exercises and metaphors for sleep.	Home practice: 10–20 min/d Log: diary of sessions and total minutes	Not reported	Not reported		Not reported
Black et al,[51] 2015	Not reported	Certified[a] mindfulness teacher with 20 y mindfulness practice	Not reported	Formal meditation: sitting, mindful eating, walking meditation, and mindful movement	Not reported	Home practice: started with 5 min/d and increased to 20 min/d by wk 6. Log: diary of number of independent sessions and total minutes	Mindfulness book, audio recordings for guided meditation	Not reported		Not reported

(continued on next page)

Table 3
(continued)

First Author, Year	Instructor Information			Mindfulness Details	Specific Sleep Instructions	Intervention Details			Participant Information
	Instruction Experience	Mindfulness Training	Clinical Qualifications			Meditation Practice/Log	Types of Materials	Monitoring of Adverse Events	Prior Experience with Meditation
Garcia et al,[52] 2018	Referred to as experienced	Not reported	Not reported	Formal meditation: seated relaxation, body scan, and breathing, breath awareness	Practice at night lying in bed just before sleeping	Home practice: varied by wk from 8–40 min, 1–3 times/d Log: when and for how long meditated	Audio recordings for guided meditation	Not reported	Not reported
Garland et al,[53] 2014; Garland et al,[54] 2015	10 + years of experience delivering MBSR	Certified[a] MBSR instructor from CFM	Nurse	Formal meditation: body scan, sitting, walking, movement, and Hatha yoga	No specific instructions were provided for sleep	Home practice: 45 min/d Log: not reported	Workbook, readings, audio recordings for guided meditation	Not reported	Excluded if they had prior experience with MBSR or CBT-I
Gross et al,[55] 2011	Not reported	Certified[a] MBSR instructor from CFM	Not reported	Formal meditation: body scan, standing, sitting, walking, and gentle yoga	Emphasized sleep and sleep stress readings from Full Catastrophe Living by Jon Kabat Zinn, which recommends breath focus in bed to reduce sleep effort	Home practice: 45 min/d at least 6 d/wk for 8 wk followed by 20 min/d for 3 mo Log: duration was tracked with electronic logger (HOBO® data logger)	Workbook, readings, audio recordings for guided meditation	Adverse events tracked and none were reported	Not reported
Nakamura et al,[58] 2011	Not reported	Certified[b] MBB instructor	Licensed clinical social worker	Focused awareness/attention exercises (no formal meditation practice)	Encouraged to practice exercises before bed	Home practice: as much as possible Log: not reported	Mind-Body map	Not reported	Not reported

Study									
Nakamura et al,[57] 2013	MBB: Not reported MM: Referred to as experienced	Certified[b] MBB instructor "Years" of meditation experience	Licensed clinical social worker Licensed clinical social worker	Focused awareness/attention exercises (no formal meditation practice) Formal meditation: sitting, walking, body scan, and awareness training	Not reported	Home practice: as much as possible Log: not reported	Mind-Body map, reference to a textbook used Copy of book "Full Catastrophe Living", audio recordings for guided meditation, handouts	Not reported	Excluded if had prior exposure to MBB, MM, MBSR, or MBCT
Nakamura et al,[56] 2017	Not reported	Certified[b] MBB instructors	Licensed clinical social workers	Focused awareness/attention exercises (no formal meditation practice)	Encouraged to practice exercises before bed and/or during the middle of night	Home practice: encouraged to practice as much as possible Log: not reported	Reference to following procedures of previous studies	Not reported	Not reported
Ong et al,[66] 2014; Ong et al,[64] 2018	MBSR: first instructor—2 y teaching experience; second instructor—15 y teaching experience MBTI: taught previous MBTI groups	MBSR: One instructor- 200 h of MBSR training MBTI: 100 h of mindfulness	MBSR: first instructor—PhD; second instructor—MD MBTI: PhD	Both groups Formal meditation: breathing, body scan, walking, and gentle yoga	None Provided additional sleep restriction and stimulus control instructions	Both groups Home practice: 30-35 min/d 6 d/wk Log: duration of meditation	Both groups A copy of book "Full Catastrophe Living", audio recordings for guided meditation, handouts	A DSMB reviewed adverse events	Not reported
Wong et al,[65] 2016; Lee et al,[63] 2018	Not reported	Referred to training but did not provide details	Registered psychologist	Formal meditation: sitting, body scan, focused attention, 3-min breathing space	Practice before going to bed, after they awoke in the morning (out of the bed) and/or any other times during the day	Home practice: 3-min breathing space 3 times/d, listen to mindfulness audio 6 d/wk Log: not reported	Audio recordings for guided meditation	Not reported	Not reported

(continued on next page)

Table 3 (continued)

First Author, Year	Instructor Information			Mindfulness Details	Intervention Details				Participant Information
	Instruction Experience	Mindfulness Training	Clinical Qualifications		Specific Sleep Instructions	Meditation Practice/Log	Types of Materials	Monitoring of Adverse Events	Prior Experience with Meditation
Wong et al,[59] 2017	2 y of experience teaching MBCT	Referred to qualified but did not provide details	Clinical psychologists	Formal meditation: eating, body scan, sitting, breathing, and walking, 3 min breathing space (80% of content was meditation)	Psychoeducation, sleep restriction and stimulus control instructions (20% of content was CBT-I)	Home practice: daily mediation practice Log: duration of meditation	Audio recordings for guided meditation	Adverse events tracked and none were reported	Not reported
Zhang, 2015	Not reported	Certified[a] MBSR instructor from CFM	Not reported	Formal meditation: sitting, standing, walking, and body scan	Not reported	Home practice: 45 min/d Log: not reported	Audio recordings for guided meditation	Not reported	Excluded if had previous contemplative, meditation, or Zen training

Abbreviations: CBT-I, cognitive behavioral therapy for insomnia; CFM, center for mindfulness; MBB, mind-body bridging; MBT, mindfulness based therapy for insomnia; MD, Doctor of Medicine; MM, mindfulness meditation; PhD, Doctor of Philosophy.

a This can range extensively from intensive programs offered at (or based on) the CFM in Medicine, Health Care, and Society at UMass Medical School to certificates provided by an online course necessitating more specific information about credentials.

b Certification requires the completion of a Mind-Body Bridging training course, which consists of approximately 40 hours of training.

recreate the intervention and test its applicability with other clinical groups in research and real-world settings. The results of this review suggest that important information about how MBTs are being applied to the treatment of insomnia and sleep disturbance is not consistently reported. This includes such information as whether people were being instructed to practice mindfulness before bed, while trying to sleep, or if they awaken during the night. This is not a small detail to overlook. Mindfulness as a practice is not specifically designed to assist with sleep onset in the same way as sleeping medication, and instruction to use it in this manner may be counterproductive. Further, mindfulness is not always conducive to the dearousal that is required to facilitate sleep, especially in the skill development stage when people may get frustrated that the processes of letting go, nonattachment, and nonreactivity do not occur as naturally or quickly as they had hoped.[34] In this way, mindfulness close to, or while in bed, may actually make the process of sleep more difficult. It is also important to note that engaging in mindfulness practice is in contrast to instruction provided by stimulus control therapy, a standard treatment recommended by the American Academy of Sleep Medicine,[69] which recommends that the bed not be paired with anything other than sleep or sex. Perhaps there are people or situations for which one method might be preferred to the other. This is yet to be determined and will continue to be so until there is a better reporting of how mindfulness is being tailored to sleep and whether it is being advocated as a bona fide first-line treatment or adjuvant to traditionally used behavioral therapies.

Recommendation 3: Identify and Measure the Specific Sleep Targets that Mindfulness-Based Therapies Are Being Used to Address

Future research is needed that moves beyond omnibus effects of MBTs for insomnia and toward the identification of mediators and moderators of treatment effects in order to better understand the process of change. The measurement of mindfulness has been criticized for being semantically ambiguous[2] yet most of the trials reviewed herein included general mindfulness measures. Mindfulness questionnaires do not consistently relate to the extent of mindfulness practice, have different response patterns in nonmeditators and those people with previous meditation experience, and may be especially influenced by social desirability.[2] Moreover, measures of mindfulness do not capture the range of putative mechanisms such as duration, frequency and setting of

mindfulness practice, acceptance, and cognitive defusion that may underly the effects of MBTs for insomnia. Given the identified problems with measuring mindfulness, a shift toward measuring empirically supported processes of change such as those hypothesized in the PPMS is recommended. Identification of these targets, along with transparent reporting of parameters of mindfulness practice, would represent a movement toward precision medicine and facilitate further testing and refinement of interventions by allowing for (1) the development of comparison interventions that are matched for nonspecific factors and (2) determining the optimal dose and setting for mindfulness practice. A similar proposal has been made in the field of health behavior change.[70] Further, defining the mechanisms may inform future work to identify potential biological processes of change.

Recommendation 4: Pay Attention to the Issue of Clinician Training and Measure Treatment Fidelity

Unlike with pharmacologic trials, nonpharmacologic treatments present difficulties due to complexity and variability of the intervention and interventionists. A meta-analysis of 46 studies with 1281 therapists and more than 14,000 patients reported that therapists account for 5% of variability in treatment outcomes.[71] Moreover, interventionist allegiance to therapies has been observed to account for 12% of variance in outcomes[72] and as much as a standardized mean difference in effect of 0.30.[73] Given the importance of therapist effects, assessing fidelity to the intervention protocol is essential to evaluate the feasibility and reproducibility of the intervention in clinical practice, as well as the true unbiased effect size. This issue is so important that it has become a recommended reporting standard for nonpharmacologic interventions.[74] This includes reporting on the credentials and training of the interventionist, as well as measuring fidelity to the principles of the intervention. More pragmatically, MBT instructors are often required to maintain their own meditation practice, which poses limits to the pool of available MBT providers and represents a potential barrier to the scalability of MBTs for insomnia.

Recommendation 5: Include Measures of Participant Expectancy and Participant Preference for Treatment

Patient expectancy and preference are at the center of pluralistic field of psychological, behavioral, and complementary therapies; however, expectancy and preference have often been overlooked as important factors influencing outcomes in randomized trials, including those in the area of sleep medicine. Matching patients with their preferred treatment has been associated with increased retention[75,76] and improved outcomes in the treatment of psychological disorders.[77,78] Patient preference is particularly important for psychological or behavioral interventions such as MBTs, which require engagement and active participation.[79] When compared with cognitive behavioral therapy for insomnia, MBSR was not inferior at the 3-month follow-up point, but only for those patients who were seeking or willing to try and persist in their assigned treatment approach.[53] This suggests that patient preferences have the potential to significantly affect treatment engagement and outcomes. Further, a recent meta-analysis demonstrated a strong expectancy/placebo effect for insomnia treatments.[80] As such, there is a need for studies that examine the role of patient preferences and expectancy in order to optimize treatment and answer important questions about how to best deliver these evidence-based interventions within the context of patient-centered care.

Recommendation 6: Avoid Assuming that Mindfulness-Based Therapies Are Devoid from the Potential for Harm and Specifically Ask About Adverse Events

Only recently have sleep researchers investigating nonpharmacologic interventions for insomnia turned their attention to possible adverse effects of treatment. Specifically, a key component of CBT-I, sleep restriction, has been associated with acute reductions in objective total sleep time, increased daytime sleepiness, and objective performance impairment in some,[81,82] but not all,[83] trials. There is a similar concern of unintended harm being raised in the area of mindfulness research. Several potential harms, including depersonalization and reexperiencing of trauma, as a result of participating in MBTs have been reported, leading the NIH to caution that "meditation could cause or worsen certain psychiatric problems."[84] It is noted in a review that only 3 trials assessed adverse events. This is an area in need of immediate attention.

SUMMARY

MBTs are increasingly being investigated as a viable treatment for insomnia or sleep disturbance. To date, 13 trials have been published since 2010 and suggest that MBTs are efficacious for improving symptoms of insomnia and sleep quality relative to psychological placebos and inactive control conditions with medium to large effects. Limited

evidence suggests that these effects are sustained at 3-month follow-up. Despite this, limited data have been collected evaluating the empirically supported mechanisms or processes of change. As such, it is unclear whether MBTs have general effects that carry over to sleep or whether they target psychological processes that specifically facilitate sleep. The collection of such information is essential to move toward personalized medicine. With this in mind, the authors propose a testable model in the PPMS that they hope will advance the next generation of research into MBTs for insomnia. In order to accomplish this goal, it is incumbent on researchers to (1) adequately detail the rationale for the MBT being offered; (2) measure the putative mechanisms or processes of change; (3) ensure that the MBT is manualized and delivered in a standardized manner; (4) report interventionist qualifications and assess potential interventionist effects; and (5) evaluate the effect of patient preference or expectation.

REFERENCES

1. Farb NAS. From retreat center to clinic to boardroom? Perils and promises of the modern mindfulness movement. Religions 2014;5(4):1062–86.
2. Van Dam NT, van Vugt MK, Vago DR, et al. Mind the hype: a critical evaluation and prescriptive agenda for research on mindfulness and meditation. Perspect Psychol Sci 2018;13(1):36–61.
3. Davidson RJ, Kaszniak AW. Conceptual and methodological issues in research on mindfulness and meditation. Am Psychol 2015;70(7):581–92.
4. Dimidjian S, Linehan MM. Defining an agenda for future research on the clinical application of mindfulness practice. Clin Psychol Sci Pract 2003;10(2):166–71.
5. Kabat-Zinn J. Full catastrophe living (revised version): using the wisdom of your body and mind to face stress, pain, and illness. New York: Bantam Books; 2013.
6. Lutz A, Jha AP, Dunne JD, et al. Investigating the phenomenological matrix of mindfulness-related practices from a neurocognitive perspective. Am Psychol 2015;70(7):632–58.
7. Borbely AA, Daan S, Wirz-Justice A, et al. The two-process model of sleep regulation: a reappraisal. J Sleep Res 2016;25(2):131–43.
8. Espie CA. Insomnia: conceptual issues in the development, persistence, and treatment of sleep disorder in adults. Annu Rev Psychol 2002;53:215–43.
9. Perlis ML, Ellis JG, Kloss JD, et al. Etiology and pathophysiology of insomnia. In: Kryger M, Roth T, Dement WC, editors. Principles and practice of sleep medicine. 6th edition. Philadelphia: Elsevier; 2017. p. 769–84.

10. Perlis ML, Giles DE, Mendelson WB, et al. Psycho-physiological insomnia: the behavioural model and a neurocognitive perspective. J Sleep Res 1997; 6(3):179–88.

11. Riemann D, Spiegelhalder K, Feige B, et al. The hyperarousal model of insomnia: a review of the concept and its evidence. Sleep Med Rev 2010; 14(1):19–31.

12. Bonnet MH, Arand DL. Hyperarousal and insomnia: state of the science. Sleep Med Rev 2010;14(1):9–15.

13. Spielman AJ, Caruso LS, Glovinsky PB. A behavioral perspective on insomnia treatment. Psychiatr Clin North Am 1987;10(4):541–53.

14. Spielman AJ, Yang C, Glovinsky PB. Assessment techniques for insomnia. In: Kryger M, Roth T, Dement WC, editors. Principles and practice of sleep medicine. 5th edition. Philadelphia: Elsevier; 2011. p. 1632–45.

15. Buysse DJ, Germain A, Hall M, et al. A neurobiological model of insomnia. Drug Discov Today Dis Models 2011;8(4):129–37.

16. Harvey AG. A cognitive model of insomnia. Behav Res Ther 2002;40(8):869–93.

17. Lundh LG, Broman JE. Insomnia as an interaction between sleep-interfering and sleep-interpreting processes. J Psychosom Res 2000;49(5):299–310.

18. Morin CM, Espie CA. Insomnia: a clinical guide to assessment and treatment. New York: Kluwer Academic; 2004.

19. Ong JC, Ulmer CS, Manber R. Improving sleep with mindfulness and acceptance: a metacognitive model of insomnia. Behav Res Ther 2012;50(11): 651–60.

20. Carney CE, Edinger JD, Morin CM, et al. Examining maladaptive beliefs about sleep across insomnia patient groups. J Psychosom Res 2010;68(1):57–65.

21. Morin CM, Stone J, Trinkle D, et al. Dysfunctional beliefs and attitudes about sleep among older adults with and without insomnia complaints. Psychol Aging 1993;8(3):463–7.

22. Harvey AG. Pre-sleep cognitive activity: a comparison of sleep-onset insomniacs and good sleepers. Br J Clin Psychol 2000;39(Pt 3):275–86.

23. Kuisk LA, Bertelson AD, Walsh JK. Presleep cognitive hyperarousal and affect as factors in objective and subjective insomnia. Percept Mot Skills 1989; 69(3 Pt 2):1219–25.

24. Broomfield NM, Espie CA. Towards a valid, reliable measure of sleep effort. J Sleep Res 2005;14(4):401–7.

25. Lundh LG. The role of acceptance and mindfulness in the treatment of insomnia. J Cogn Psychother 2005;19(1):29–39.

26. Harvey AG. I can't sleep, my mins is racing! an investigation of strategies of thought control in insomnia. Behav Cogn Psychother 2001;29(1):3–11.

27. Nicassio PM, Mendlowitz DR, Fussell JJ, et al. The phenomenology of the pre-sleep state: the development of the pre-sleep arousal scale. Behav Res Ther 1985;23(3):263–71.

28. Taylor DJ, Lichstein KL, Durrence HH, et al. Epidemiology of insomnia, depression, and anxiety. Sleep 2005;28(11):1457–64.

29. Thomsen DK, Mehlsen MY, Christensen S, et al. Rumination—relationship with negative mood and sleep quality. Personality and Individual Differences 2003;34(7):1293–301.

30. Carney CE, Edinger JD, Meyer B, et al. Symptom-focused rumination and sleep disturbance. Behav Sleep Med 2006;4(4):228–41.

31. Hayes SC, Luoma JB, Bond FW, et al. Acceptance and commitment therapy: model, processes and outcomes. Behav Res Ther 2006;44(1):1–25.

32. Hayes SC, Villatte M, Levin M, et al. Open, aware, and active: contextual approaches as an emerging trend in the behavioral and cognitive therapies. Annu Rev Clin Psychol 2011;7:141–68.

33. McCracken LM, Williams JL, Tang NKY. Psychological flexibility may reduce insomnia in persons with chronic pain: a preliminary retrospective study. Pain Med 2011;12(6):904–12.

34. Lundh LG. Insomnia. In: McCracken LM, editor. Mindfulness and acceptacne in behavioral medicine: current theory and practice. Oakland (CA): New Harbinger; 2011. p. 131–58.

35. McCracken LM, Vowles KE. Acceptance and commitment therapy and mindfulness for chronic pain: model, process, and progress. Am Psychol 2014;69(2):178–87.

36. Harvey AG, Buysse DJ. Treating sleep problems: a transdiagnostic approach. New York: Guilford Publications; 2017.

37. Riemann D. Insomnia and comorbid psychiatric disorders. Sleep Med 2007;8(Suppl 4):S15–20.

38. Taylor DJ, Mallory LJ, Lichstein KL, et al. Comorbidity of chronic insomnia with medical problems. Sleep 2007;30(2):213–8.

39. Daly-Eichenhardt A, Scott W, Howard-Jones M, et al. Changes in sleep problems and psychological flexibility following interdisciplinary acceptance and commitment therapy for chronic pain: an observational cohort study. Front Psychol 2016;7:1326.

40. Gong H, Ni CX, Liu YZ, et al. Mindfulness meditation for insomnia: a meta-analysis of randomized controlled trials. J Psychosom Res 2016;89:1–6.

41. Haller H, Winkler MM, Klose P, et al. Mindfulness-based interventions for women with breast cancer: an updated systematic review and meta-analysis. Acta Oncol 2017;56(12):1665–76.

42. American Psychiatry Association A. Diagnostic and statistical manual of mental disorders: DSM-IV. Washington, DC: American Psychiatry Association; 1994.

43. Association ASD. The international classification of sleep disorders: diagnostic and coding manual.

2nd edition. New York: American Sleep Disorders Association; 2005.

44. Hays RD, Martin SA, Sesti AM, et al. Psychometric properties of the medical outcomes study sleep measure. Sleep Med 2005;6(1):41–4.

45. Buysse DJ, Reynolds CF 3rd, Monk TH, et al. The Pittsburgh sleep quality index: a new instrument for psychiatric practice and research. Psychiatry Res 1989;28(2):193–213.

46. Yates SL, Morley S, Eccleston C, et al. A scale for rating the quality of psychological trials for pain. Pain 2005;117(3):314–25.

47. Lipsey MW, Wilson DB. Practical meta-analysis. Thousand Oaks (CA): Sage Publications, Inc; 2001.

48. Higgins JP, Green S. Cochrane handbook for systematic reviews of interventions. Wiley Online Library: Cochrane Collaboration; 2008.

49. Orwin RG. A fail-safe N for effect size in meta-analysis. Journal of Educational Statistics 1983;8(2):157–9.

50. Higgins JP, Thompson SG. Quantifying heterogeneity in a meta-analysis. Stat Med 2002;21(11):1539–58.

51. Black DS, O'Reilly GA, Olmstead R, et al. Mindfulness meditation and improvement in sleep quality and daytime impairment among older adults with sleep disturbances: a randomized clinical trial. JAMA Intern Med 2015;175(4):494–501.

52. Garcia MC, Kozasa EH, Tufik S, et al. The effects of mindfulness and relaxation training for insomnia (MRTI) on postmenopausal women: a pilot study. Menopause 2018;25(9):992–1003.

53. Garland SN, Carlson LE, Stephens AJ, et al. Mindfulness-based stress reduction compared with cognitive behavioral therapy for the treatment of insomnia comorbid with cancer: a randomized, partially blinded, noninferiority trial. J Clin Oncol 2014;32(5):449–57.

54. Garland SN, Rouleau CR, Campbell T, et al. The comparative impact of mindfulness-based cancer recovery (MBCR) and cognitive behavior therapy for insomnia (CBT-I) on sleep and mindfulness in cancer patients. Explore (NY) 2015;11(6):445–54.

55. Gross CR, Kreitzer MJ, Reilly-Spong M, et al. Mindfulness-based stress reduction versus pharmacotherapy for chronic primary insomnia: a randomized controlled clinical trial. Explore (NY) 2011;7(2):76–87.

56. Nakamura Y, Lipschitz DL, Donaldson GW, et al. Investigating clinical benefits of a novel sleep-focused mind-body program on gulf war illness symptoms: a randomized controlled trial. Psychosom Med 2017;79(6):706–18.

57. Nakamura Y, Lipschitz DL, Kuhn R, et al. Investigating efficacy of two brief mind-body intervention programs for managing sleep disturbance in cancer survivors: a pilot randomized controlled trial. J Cancer Surviv 2013;7(2):165–82.

58. Nakamura Y, Lipschitz DL, Landward R, et al. Two sessions of sleep-focused mind-body bridging improve self-reported symptoms of sleep and PTSD in veterans: a pilot randomized controlled trial. J Psychosom Res 2011;70(4):335–45.

59. Wong SY, Zhang DX, Li CC, et al. Comparing the effects of mindfulness-based cognitive therapy and sleep psycho-education with exercise on chronic insomnia: a randomised controlled trial. Psychother Psychosom 2017;86(4):241–53.

60. Amutio A, Franco C, Sanchez-Sanchez LC, et al. Effects of mindfulness training on sleep problems in patients with fibromyalgia. Front Psychol 2018;9:1365.

61. deok Baik K. Evaluating acceptance and commitment therapy for insomnia: a randomized controlled trial. Bowling Green (OH): Bowling Green State University; 2015.

62. Zhang JX, Liu XH, Xie XH, et al. Mindfulness-based stress reduction for chronic insomnia in adults older than 75 years: a randomized, controlled, single-blind clinical trial. Explore (NY) 2015;11(3):180–5.

63. Lee CW, Ree MJ, Wong MY. Effective insomnia treatments: investigation of processes in mindfulness and cognitive therapy. Behav Change 2018;35(2):1–20.

64. Ong JC, Xia Y, Smith-Mason CE, et al. A randomized controlled trial of mindfulness meditation for chronic insomnia: effects on daytime symptoms and cognitive-emotional arousal. Mindfulness 2018;9(6):1–11.

65. Wong MY, Ree MJ, Lee CW. Enhancing CBT for chronic insomnia: a randomised clinical trial of additive components of mindfulness or cognitive therapy. Clin Psychol Psychother 2016;23(5):377–85.

66. Ong JC, Manber R, Segal Z, et al. A randomized controlled trial of mindfulness meditation for chronic insomnia. Sleep 2014;37(9):1553–63.

67. Ong JC. Mindfulness-based therapy for insomnia. Washington, DC: American Psychological Association; 2017.

68. Dalrymple KL, Fiorentino L, Politi MC, et al. Incorporating principles from acceptance and commitment therapy into cognitive-behavioral therapy for insomnia: a case example. J Contemp Psychother 2010;40(4):209–17.

69. Morgenthaler T, Kramer M, Alessi C, et al. Practice parameters for the psychological and behavioral treatment of insomnia: an update. An American Academy of Sleep Medicine Report. Sleep 2006;29(11):1415–9.

70. Sheeran P, Klein WM, Rothman AJ. Health behavior change: moving from observation to intervention. Annu Rev Psychol 2017;68:573–600.

71. Baldwin SA, Imel ZE. Therapist effects: findings and methods. 5th edition. Hoboken (NJ): Wiley; 2013.

72. Munder T, Flückiger C, Gerger H, et al. Is the allegiance effect an epiphenomenon of true efficacy

differences between treatments? A meta-analysis. J Couns Psychol 2012;59(4):631–7.

73. Falkenstrom F, Markowitz JC, Jonker H, et al. Can psychotherapists function as their own controls? Meta-analysis of the crossed therapist design in comparative psychotherapy trials. J Clin Psychiatry 2013;74(5):482–91.

74. Boutron I, Moher D, Altman DG, et al. Extending the CONSORT statement to randomized trials of non-pharmacologic treatment: explanation and elaboration. Ann Intern Med 2008;148(4):295–309.

75. Sidani S, Bootzin RR, Epstein DR, et al. Attrition in randomized and preference trials of behavioural treatments for insomnia. Can J Nurs Res 2015; 47(1):17–34.

76. Steidtmann D, Manber R, Arnow BA, et al. Patient treatment preference as a predictor of response and attrition in treatment for chronic depression. Depress Anxiety 2012;29(10):896–905.

77. McHugh RK, Whitton SW, Peckham AD, et al. Patient preference for psychological vs pharmacologic treatment of psychiatric disorders: a meta-analytic review. J Clin Psychiatry 2013;74(6):595–602.

78. Williams R, Farquharson L, Palmer L, et al. Patient preference in psychological treatment and associations with self-reported outcome: national cross-sectional survey in England and Wales. BMC Psychiatry 2016;16:4.

79. Kowalski CJ, Mrdjenovich AJ. Patient preference clinical trials: why and when they will sometimes be preferred. Perspect Biol Med 2013;56(1):18–35.

80. Yeung V, Sharpe L, Glozier N, et al. A systematic review and meta-analysis of placebo versus no treatment for insomnia symptoms. Sleep Med Rev 2018;38:17–27.

81. Kyle SD, Miller CB, Rogers Z, et al. Sleep restriction therapy for insomnia is associated with reduced objective total sleep time, increased daytime somnolence, and objectively impaired vigilance: implications for the clinical management of insomnia disorder. Sleep 2014;37(2): 229–37.

82. Kyle SD, Morgan K, Spiegelhalder K, et al. No pain, no gain: an exploratory within-subjects mixed-methods evaluation of the patient experience of sleep restriction therapy (SRT) for insomnia. Sleep Med 2011;12(8):735–47.

83. Whittall H, Pillion M, Gradisar M. Daytime sleepiness, driving performance, reaction time and inhibitory control during sleep restriction therapy for Chronic Insomnia Disorder. Sleep Med 2018;45: 44–8.

84. Health NCfCal. Meditatin: In depth. 2017; NCCIH Pub No.: D308. Available at: https://nccih.nih.gov/ health/meditation/overview.htm#hed5. Accessed October 10, 2018.

Brief Behavioral Treatment of Insomnia

Heather E. Gunn, PhD[a],*, Joshua Tutek, MA[a], Daniel J. Buysse, MD[b]

KEYWORDS

- Insomnia • Behavioral treatment • Brief treatment • BBTI

KEY POINTS

- Cognitive behavioral treatment for insomnia (CBTI) is an effective treatment of insomnia; however, there are insufficient CBTI providers for the 10% to 25% of the population who have insomnia.
- Brief behavioral treatment for insomnia (BBTI) is a 4-session manualized treatment paradigm administrable in medical settings by nonpsychologist health professionals.
- BBTI is effective in reducing symptoms of insomnia, such as sleep onset latency, wake after sleep onset, and sleep efficiency. In some cases, BBTI resulted in full remission from insomnia.
- Ongoing clinical trials are further testing the efficacy of BBTI in alternative treatment deliveries (video conference) and in primary medical care settings.

INTRODUCTION

Insomnia is defined by difficulty with sleep initiation, sleep maintenance, and daytime impairment in social, educational, or other areas of functioning.[1] It is the most common sleep disorder, with prevalence in the general population ranging from 10% to 25%.[2] Individuals with insomnia symptoms have high health care utilization and costs and increased workplace absenteeism and reduced productivity.[3] Insomnia is often managed with hypnotics, which are efficacious, but also pose risks for side effects, dependence, and withdrawal symptoms.[4] Cognitive behavioral treatment of insomnia (CBTI) is an effective treatment of insomnia and is recommended as the initial treatment by the American College of Physicians.[5,6]

Despite favorable results, CBTI can be impractical as a first line of treatment. Specialists in behavioral sleep medicine often administer CBTI over a relatively long duration (6–8 sessions). As such, there is a significant discrepancy between the number of people who would benefit from CBTI treatment and the number of CBTI providers. Moreover, individuals with insomnia have psychiatric and medical comorbidities and are more likely to present with their sleep complaints to a general practitioner.[7] To extend the reach of behavioral treatments for insomnia to those with comorbidities and to other medical settings, Buysse and colleagues[8,9] developed a brief, manualized protocol administrable in medical settings, *brief behavioral treatment for insomnia* (BBTI). In a 2011 initial efficacy study, individuals who completed BBTI demonstrated improvement in sleep over 6 months.[9] The authors provide a brief overview of BBTI, review its efficacy in varied populations, discuss limitations, and make suggestions for future research using BBTI.

BRIEF BEHAVIORAL TREATMENT FOR INSOMNIA OVERVIEW

BBTI was developed to be brief, acceptable to patients taking medications and with other

Disclosure Statement: H.E. Gunn and J. Tutek have no financial disclosures to report. D.J. Buysse has served as a paid consultant to BeHealth Solutions, Emmi Solutions, and Bayer HealthCare (last 3 years).
[a] Department of Psychology, University of Alabama, 505 Hackberry Lane, Box 870348, Tuscaloosa, AL 35487-0348, USA; [b] Sleep & Chronobiology Center, Department of Psychiatry, University of Pittsburgh, 3811 O'Hara Street, Pittsburgh, PA 15213, USA
* Corresponding author.
E-mail address: hegunn@ua.edu

sleep.theclinics.com

comorbidities, and efficacious in a short time period. It is deliverable by professionals with minimal specialty training (the initial efficacy trial was delivered by a nurse practitioner with no prior sleep medicine or behavioral interventions). The design targets 2 physiologic processes that regulate sleep: Homeostatic drive that increases sleep propensity as duration of wakefulness increases, and circadian drive that governs 24-hour rhythms in sleep-wake propensity. Treatment focuses on modifying sleep behaviors that influence homeostatic and circadian sleep regulation. In particular, the duration of daytime wakefulness is increased to optimize sleep drive, and sleep timing is regulated to establish consistent cues for circadian entrainment.[5,6]

Table 1 presents a brief summary and rationale of the protocol, which is described in more detail in later discussion. For a more detailed overview, see Troxel and colleagues.[8] The primary components of BBTI are stimulus control[10] and sleep restriction,[11] which are behaviorally focused modifications with strong empirical support for improving insomnia symptoms. These techniques minimize "psychological" concepts that can be challenging to address in medical environments. Before treatment, patients complete a clinical interview, standardized questionnaires for sleep and daytime symptoms, and 1 to 2 weeks of sleep diaries, which facilitate individualized treatment recommendations. The original protocol consists of 2 in-person meetings (sessions 1 and 3) and 2 telephone check-ins (sessions 2 and 4).

Session 1 (45–75 minutes) introduces most of the intervention components, including health sleep practices, the 2-process model of sleep regulation, and treatment recommendations. An interactive workbook guides session 1, beginning with a review of behaviors that help or hinder sleep and an overview of the interplay between the homeostatic and circadian drives in regulating sleep. This education informs the rationale for specific behavioral recommendations to limit time in bed and maintain a consistent wake time (**Fig. 1** represents one workbook page). The therapist and patient then use the workbook to calculate and record average sleep parameters from sleep diaries to facilitate insight into day-to-day sleep-impairing practices. Finally, the therapist introduces the patient to the "Four Rules" to improve sleep, relating these rules to the physiologic sleep-regulatory mechanisms, basic behavioral conditioning principles, and the patient's individual sleep characteristics on diaries (see **Table 1**).

The patient and therapist brainstorm distracting, low-stimulation activities that can be pursued in dim lighting while the patient is outside of the bedroom and unable to sleep. With guidance from the therapist, a new sleep schedule is established in which the patient selects a consistent wakeup time and works backward to determine bedtime. Session 1 concludes with a customized "sleep prescription" that includes the target daily bed and wake time, nighttime out-of-bed activities, recommendations for medication timing and dosage, if applicable, and scheduling of follow-up sessions. Troxel and colleagues[5] note that acknowledging the anticipated difficulty of adhering to the prescription during this time is useful for setting realistic expectations for patients and enhancing their compliance to treatment.

Session 2 is a follow-up phone call (<20 minutes) regarding the patient's current sleep and daytime functioning status as well as any noticed changes. The therapist confirms adherence to sleep recommendations, provides support, and engages the patient in problem solving. The patient has their sleep diary on hand to facilitate review of the week's data; however, a night-by-night review of the week's sleep is not required.

Session 3 (30 minutes) is an in-person meeting to review progress and address difficulties with recommendations, monitor and reinforce adherence, and provide instructions for titrating sleep schedule. The patient is instructed to maintain changes to the sleep schedule for the next week. Patients are instructed to follow the algorithm of sleep extension or restriction (see **Table 1**) on a weekly basis throughout treatment, and beyond treatment discontinuation if sleep problems persist.

Session 4 (<20 minutes) is a final phone call to discuss progress and treatment challenges, increase time in bed as needed, and review relapse prevention. The 4 rules for better sleep and the instructions for increasing or decreasing time in bed are also readdressed. It is also useful to discuss scenarios or periods during which patients will likely encounter increased sleep disturbance, which may aid in developing preemptive strategies to prevent relapse during challenging periods.

UPDATE ON BRIEF BEHAVIORAL TREATMENT FOR INSOMNIA EFFICACY

The goals of BBTI are similar to other insomnia treatment modalities: (1) improve sleep quality and quantity and (2) reduce daytime impairment.[1] Improvements in these domains are generally assessed using questionnaires addressing sleep quality (eg, Pittsburgh sleep quality index; PSQI),[12] insomnia severity (eg, insomnia severity index; ISI),[13] and daily sleep diaries in which patients estimate and record their bedtime, sleep

Table 1
Brief behavioral treatment for insomnia session-by-session methods and rationale

Session	Method	Rationale
Pretreatment		
Sleep evaluation	Clinical interview with provider	Sleep diagnosis and rule out other sleep disorders
Questionnaires	Baseline measures of sleep quality (eg, PSQI) and insomnia severity (eg, ISI), sleepiness (eg, ESS)	Determines nature and severity of patient impairment in sleep and daytime functioning[31]
Sleep diaries	Two weeks daily sleep diaries (eg, bedtime, wake time, etc.)	Accurately estimate sleep pattern[32]; facilitate personalized sleep schedule[11]
Session 1 (45–75 min)		
Healthy sleep practices	Patient is educated on practices that facilitate sleep (eg, dim evening light), or hinder sleep (eg, computer in bed)	Distinguish healthy sleep practices from active components of treatment[8,33]
Two-process model of sleep regulation[34]	1. Homeostatic sleep drive (sleep propensity increases with the duration of wakefulness) 2. Circadian sleep drive (sleep propensity governed by 24-h biological pacemaker)	Behavioral recommendations for sleep harness and strengthen components of 2-process model[8]
Four sleep rules:	1. Reduce time in bed (usual TST + 30 min, never reduce TIB below 6 h) 2. Establish consistent wake time 3. Go to bed when sleepy 4. Get out of bed when not sleeping in 30 min	1. ↑ Homeostatic sleep drive; ↓ sleep latency[11] 2. Strengthen circadian signaling[10]; ↓ chance of phase delay[35]; ↑ homeostatic sleep drive[11] 3. ↑ Homeostatic sleep drive[11]; ↑ awareness of internal cues of sleepiness[10] 4. Facilitates reconditioning to associate bed with sleep[36]
Session 2 (<20 min)		
Phone follow-up	Review patient's sleep quality, diaries, daytime functioning, and adherence to recommendations and schedule prescribed at session 1	Provide interim support, identify specific challenges to adherence, and problem solve for solutions[8]
Session 3 (30 min)		
In-person follow-up	Therapist and patient review progress, address challenges, and reinforce adherence	
Sleep schedule titration	Adjust sleep schedule as needed: • If SOL and WASO <30 min on most nights, add 15 min to time in bed (advance bedtime or delay wake time). • If SOL or WASO >30 min on most nights, decrease time in bed by 15 min	Sleep schedule should facilitate patient's core sleep requirement and maximize SE and homeostatic drive[11]

(continued on next page)

Session	Method	Rationale
Table 1 *(continued)*		
Session 4 (<20 min)		
Phone follow-up	Review progress, address challenges, monitor and reinforce adherence to recommendations Titrate as needed; TIB is *decreased* when sleep is poor and *increased* when sleep is good	
Relapse prevention	Therapist and patient anticipate insomnia recurrence (eg, stressful events at work or home). Review recommendations for sleep titration	Minimize perpetuating factors in insomnia[37]; develop proactive strategies to mitigate relapse[8]

onset latency (SOL), wake after sleep onset (WASO), wake time, and out-of-bed time. Daily diary estimates can then be used to estimate total in bed (TIB), total sleep time (TST), and sleep efficiency (SE), which is expressed as the percent of time the patient was in bed asleep (ie, SE = TST/TIB * 100). SOL, WASO, and SE can also be derived from actigraphy and polysomnography (PSG). Insomnia treatments, including BBTI, are evaluated by their ability to decrease scores on one or more of these global rating scales or specific sleep parameters. Although PSG is the "gold standard" for sleep assessment, it is not indicated in the evaluation of insomnia.[1] Use of PSG to evaluate insomnia is also less common than daily diaries or actigraphy due to participant burden and cost. Finally, the efficacy of BBTI (and other treatments for insomnia) can be described by a priori operationalized definitions of response to treatment and remittance of symptoms.

Results from 6 studies using BBTI to treat insomnia are outlined in **Table 2**. Study designs were either randomized controlled trials (RCTs; 4) or one-group quasiexperimental designs (2). Sample sizes ranged from 10 to 79 individuals. Study samples were diverse in terms of age, comorbidities (eg, human immunodeficiency virus),[14] medical history (eg, cancer survivors),[15] and insomnia

Rule 1: Reduce your time in bed

- Cutting down your time in bed = increasing how long you've been awake
- Being awake longer leads to quicker, deeper, more solid sleep
- Not decreasing the amount of SLEEP you get, just the amount of AWAKE time in bed
- How long in bed? <u>Sleep</u> time + 30 minutes

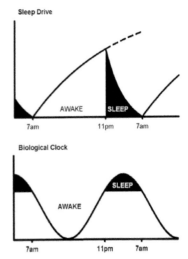

Fig. 1. BBTI workbook page with description of first "rule" of treatment on the left and a depiction of the 2-process model of sleep on the right. The therapist and the patient review the rules and the rationale together.

Table 2
Results from studies using brief behavioral treatment for insomnia for treatment of insomnia

First Author, y	Sample	Study Design	Sleep Measures	Efficacy Criteria	Efficacy and Other Sleep Outcomes
Germain et al,[16] 2006	N = 35, 71% women, M age = 70.2 ± 6.4 y	RCT BBTI vs information control	PSQI, diary SOL, TST, WASO, SE	Response = 3 pt decrease on PSQI or 10% increase in SE; Remission = response + PSQI <5 or SE >85%	BBTI group: 71% response and 53% remission; control group: 39% response and 17% remission. Other sleep outcomes: BBTI improvements in diary and PSQI > than control
Buysse et al,[9] 2011	N = 79, 70% women, M age = 71.7	RCT BBTI vs information control	PSQI, ESS, diary, actigraphy, & PSG SOL, TST, WASO, SE	Response = 3 pt decrease on PSQI or 10% increase in diary SE; remission = response + PSQI <5 or SE >85%; no insomnia diagnosis based on structured clinical interview	BBTI group: 55% no longer met insomnia criteria, 40% response, and 25% remission; control group: 13% no longer met insomnia criteria, 20% response, and <5% remission. Other sleep outcomes: BBTI improvements in PSQI, diary SOL, WASO, & SE > than control; BBTI improvements in actigraphy SOL, WASO, & SE > control; BBTI actigraphy TST < control; no PSG group differences
Wang et al,[38] 2016	N = 79 adults with treatment resistant insomnia, 54% women, M age = 41.6 ± 8.42	RCT BBTI vs sleep hygiene	PSQI, ESS, DBAS, ISI, diary SOL, TIB, SE, WASO	Not specified	BBTI improvements in PSQI, ESS, DBAS, ISI, diary SOL, TIB, SE, WASO > control group

(continued on next page)

Table 2
(continued)

First Author, y	Sample	Study Design	Sleep Measures	Efficacy Criteria	Efficacy and Other Sleep Outcomes
Buchanan et al,[14] 2018	N = 12 adults with HIV, 77.3% men, M age = 46 (range 30–59)	One-group quasi-experimental pilot	PSQI, ISI, diary SOL WASO, SQ, PROMIS-sleep impairment	Not specified	↓ PSQI, ISI, PROMIS diary SOL, WASO, & SQ (lower score = better sleep quality), ↑ SE Other sleep outcomes: ISI scores decreased to no "clinically important insomnia," ↑ TST
Zhou et al,[15] 2017	N = 10 adolescent and young adult cancer survivors, 60% women, M age = 28.1 ± 7.2	Modified BBTI, one-group quasiexperimental	PSQI, ISI, diary TST, & SE	Not specified	↓ PSQI, ISI, diary SOL & WASO ↑ diary SE
McCrae et al,[17] 2018	N = 62, 42% women, M age = 69.4 ± 7.7	RCT BBTI vs self-monitoring control	Diary SQ, diary & actigraphy SOL, TST, WASO, SE	Response = ≥10% in SE, remit = response criteria, + SE ≥85% + SQ ≥2.5	BBTI group: 53% response and 28% remit; control group: 13% response and 7% response Other sleep outcomes: BBTI improvements in diary SOL, WASO, SE, & SQ > than control group; no differences between BBTI and control group on actigraphy outcomes

Abbreviations: DBAS, dysfunctional beliefs about sleep; ESS, Epworth sleepiness scale; M, Mean; PROMIS, patient-reported outcomes measurement information system; pt, patient; SQ, sleep quality.

medication use. Three studies found better response and remissions rates in BBTI groups compared with information or self-monitoring control groups.[9,16,17] Results from 4 studies indicated that improvements in diary-assessed sleep quality, SOL, WASO, and SE were greater in BBTI groups than in a control condition. Buysse and colleagues[9] found that improvements in actigraphy-assessed SOL, WASO, and SE were greater in the BBTI group compared with the control condition. In contrast, McCrae and colleagues[17] found no group differences in actigraphy-assessed sleep outcomes. Only one study reported on pre-post PSG assessments and found no pre-post or group differences in PSG-assessed sleep.[9] All studies reported postintervention improvements in sleep diary measures. Two studies demonstrated sustained improvements. McCrae and colleagues[17] found that improvements in diary-assessed SOL, WASO, and SE were sustained at 3 months. Among 25 BBTI recipients at 6 months after treatment, 40% met criteria for remission, 44% met criteria for response, and 64% no longer met diagnostic criteria for insomnia.[9] BBTI also appears to be acceptable in terms of treatment adherence outcomes, in keeping with protocol aims. Participants in a BBTI treatment group restricted their time in bed as instructed and were 80% to 90% adherent to sleep hygiene and stimulus control recommendations.[17]

Thus, results from existing studies on BBTI demonstrate that it is acceptable and efficacious in improving both global and specific symptoms of insomnia assessed via daily diary (ie, SOL, WASO, SE). In some studies, patients no longer met criteria for insomnia. However, response to treatment may vary depending on individual differences in sleep, mental health, and other comorbidities. For example, Troxel and colleagues[18] found that patients with *more* anxious and depressive symptoms at baseline were more likely to demonstrate an a priori–defined treatment response to BBTI (≥3-point change in PSQI score or ≥10% change in SE). Longer sleep durations at baseline were also associated with more likelihood of a treatment response, whereas individuals with short sleep durations at baseline were less likely to respond to BBTI treatment.[18]

Treatment response may also vary depending on medical comorbidities, especially those that influence nighttime sleep behavior. Older adults with nocturia had reduced BBTI treatment effects compared with older adults without nocturia.[19] To the authors' knowledge, no other studies have examined predictors of treatment response. Based on the existing literature, BBTI appears to be efficacious in older adults with diverse medical

histories, but treatment response may be attenuated based on individual differences in medical comorbidities, sleep duration, and distress at baseline.

OTHER IMPLICATIONS OF BRIEF BEHAVIORAL TREATMENT FOR INSOMNIA

Improving or resolving insomnia has a positive impact on other medical and psychological domains. For example, individuals who underwent CBTI had reduced pain ratings after treatment even though pain management was not a part of the treatment protocol.[20] Similarly, Manber and colleagues[21] found that individuals with major depression and insomnia had better depression remission rates when they were offered CBTI in addition to pharmaceutical treatment of depression. Buysse and colleagues[9] found that individuals in the BBTI group had improved scores on measures of depression and general health, but not anxiety, compared with the control group. However, McCrae and colleagues[17] found no differences in mood and anxiety in response to BBTI. Although BBTI was not associated with improved cognitive performance at 4 or 12 weeks after treatment compared with the control condition, improved sleep (across groups) was associated with small performance improvements.[17,22] However, BBTI is associated with improvements in medical outcomes. In a secondary analysis of a BBTI trial,[9] Tyagi and colleagues[23] examined whether BBTI was associated with changes in self-reported nocturia (excessive nighttime voids). Nocturnal voids decreased in the BBTI and *increased* in the control group.

The brevity and flexibility of BBTI facilitates dissemination via varied treatment deliveries and to populations with comorbidities. For example, in an RCT, BBTI was adapted to include a focus on military factors that contribute to symptoms of insomnia in military veterans (BBTI-MV).[24] The BBTI-MV group had a greater response to treatment compared with the control group (76% vs 50%, respectively), although this difference was not statistically significant. In a small sample of cancer survivors, Zhou and colleagues[15] piloted the efficacy of a BBTI protocol that was modified to include components of CBTI. As presented in **Table 2**, they found that their protocol (delivered in person or via video conference) was associated with improvements in sleep quality, insomnia severity, and SOL. The efficacy of BBTI among individuals with hypertension and insomnia is currently being evaluated in an ongoing RCT, hypertension with unsatisfactory sleep health (HUSH).[25] In this large trial (the enrollment target is 625 adults), BBTI is delivered in person via Web-interface/telehealth and is compared with a self-guided Internet protocol condition (SHUTi [Sleep Healthy Using the Internet]) and an enhanced usual care condition. Results from this trial will demonstrate the effectiveness of low-cost insomnia interventions with potential for dissemination to medical settings.[25]

LIMITATIONS AND FUTURE DIRECTIONS OF BRIEF BEHAVIORAL TREATMENT FOR INSOMNIA

Much of what is known about BBTI's efficacy has been observed in older adult populations. Insomnia with comorbidities is common in older adults,[26] who are also at increased risk for side effects from medications.[27] Thus, results of BBTI trials demonstrate positive outcomes for a population most likely to benefit from a brief behavioral intervention for insomnia that is deliverable by health practitioners in a medical setting. However, evaluation on generalizability of BBTI efficacy is currently limited to 4 RCTs (in older adults) and 2 quasiexperimental designs. Results from studies on BBTI in other age ranges and comorbidities, and in other settings, are necessary.

To the authors' knowledge, there are 2 ongoing BBTI trials. In addition to the HUSH trial described above, Bramoweth and colleagues[28] are comparing the efficacy of BBTI to CBTI in Veterans Affairs primary care settings. The aims of this study are to directly compare BBTI to the "gold standard," CBTI, and to identify provider level barriers to implementation of behavioral treatment of insomnia in a primary care setting. Findings from these BBTI trials[25,28] will determine the extent to which BBTI is effective when delivered via other modalities (video/telehealth) and across medical settings (eg, primary care). Positive outcomes have the potential to reduce health care costs due to insomnia. For example, brief CBTI (a treatment paradigm similar to BBTI) was associated with reduced health care usage and a significant reduction in office visit–related costs.[29] Insomnia treatment delivered in a group format is successful[30] and may facilitate cost reduction. To the authors' knowledge, BBTI has not yet been tested in a group treatment paradigm; however, BBTI is being delivered via video/telephone conference in the HUSH trial. Treatments with few or no office visits may also facilitate cost reduction. Current and future studies will help determine whether BBTI is as effective at a reduced cost to the patient.

In addition to exploring reductions in health care usage and costs, it will be useful to determine whether BBTI is associated with other downstream psychological and health benefits. Thus far, BBTI is not directly related to cognitive improvement in one study where it was examined; however, it will be important to consider other types of cognitive assessment (eg, computerized testing paradigms) and that improvements in cognition may not be immediately apparent.[22,29] Likewise, it will be useful to continue to explore whether BBTI contributes to improved symptoms of mood and anxiety disorders. Thus far, the data are mixed; however, extended follow-up may be useful in assessing psychological outcomes.

In sum, BBTI is effective in reducing symptoms of insomnia, and in many cases, predicts insomnia remission. Treatment is successful when administered by a nonpsychologist,[9] which suggests that with some sleep education, health practitioners could effectively increase treatment availability. Individuals with varied medical histories show improvement after BBTI treatment. Ongoing and future studies will test alternate treatment deliveries (eg, video conference) and efficacy in primary care settings, which will provide further evidence of BBTI's ability to reduce insomnia across medical settings.

REFERENCES

1. Schutte-Rodin S, Broch L, Buysse D, et al. Clinical guideline for the evaluation and management of chronic insomnia in adults. J Clin Sleep Med 2008;4(5):487–504.
2. Ohayon MM. Epidemiology of insomnia: what we know and what we still need to learn. Sleep Med Rev 2002;6(2):97–111.
3. Rosekind MR, Gregory KB. Insomnia risks and costs: health, safety, and quality of life. Am J Manag Care 2010;16(8):617–26.
4. Kripke DF, Langer RD, Kline LE. Hypnotics' association with mortality or cancer: a matched cohort study. BMJ Open 2012;2(1):e000850.
5. Qaseem A, Kansagara D, Forciea MA, et al, Clinical Guidelines Committee of the American College of Physicians. Management of chronic insomnia disorder in adults: a clinical practice guideline from the American College of Physicians. Ann Intern Med 2016;165(2):125–33.
6. Trauer JM, Qian MY, Doyle JS, et al. Cognitive behavioral therapy for chronic insomnia: a systematic review and meta-analysis. Ann Intern Med 2015;163(3):191–204.
7. Espie CA, Inglis SJ, Tessier S, et al. The clinical effectiveness of cognitive behaviour therapy for chronic insomnia: implementation and evaluation of a sleep clinic in general medical practice. Behav Res Ther 2001;39(1):45–60.

8. Troxel WM, Germain A, Buysse DJ. Clinical management of insomnia with brief behavioral treatment (BBTI). Behav Sleep Med 2012;10(4):266–79.
9. Buysse DJ, Germain A, Moul DE, et al. Efficacy of brief behavioral treatment for chronic insomnia in older adults. Arch Intern Med 2011;171(10):887–95.
10. Bootzin RR, Epstein D, Wood JM. Stimulus control instructions. In: Hauri PJ, editor. Case studies in insomnia. New York: Plenum Publishing Corporation; 1991. p. 19–28.
11. Spielman AJ, Saskin P, Thorpy MJ. Treatment of chronic insomnia by restriction of time in bed. Sleep 1987;10(1):45–56.
12. Buysse DJ, Reynolds CF 3rd, Monk TH, et al. The Pittsburgh Sleep Quality Index: a new instrument for psychiatric practice and research. Psychiatry Res 1989;28(2):193–213.
13. Bastien CH, Vallieres A, Morin CM. Validation of the Insomnia Severity Index as an outcome measure for insomnia research. Sleep Med 2001;2(4):297–307.
14. Buchanan DT, McCurry SM, Eilers K, et al. Brief behavioral treatment for insomnia in persons living with HIV. Behav Sleep Med 2018;16(3):244–58.
15. Zhou ES, Vrooman LM, Manley PE, et al. Adapted delivery of cognitive-behavioral treatment for insomnia in adolescent and young adult cancer survivors: a pilot study. Behav Sleep Med 2017;15(4):288–301.
16. Germain A, Moul DE, Franzen PL, et al. Effects of a brief behavioral treatment for late-life insomnia: preliminary findings. J Clin Sleep Med 2006;2(4):403–6.
17. McCrae CS, Curtis AF, Williams JM, et al. Efficacy of brief behavioral treatment for insomnia in older adults: examination of sleep, mood, and cognitive outcomes. Sleep Med 2018;51:153–66.
18. Troxel WM, Conrad TS, Germain A, et al. Predictors of treatment response to brief behavioral treatment of insomnia (BBTI) in older adults. J Clin Sleep Med 2013;9(12):1281–9.
19. Tyagi S, Resnick NM, Perera S, et al. Behavioral treatment of chronic insomnia in older adults: does nocturia matter? Sleep 2014;37(4):681–7.
20. Vitiello MV, Rybarczyk B, Von Korff M, et al. Cognitive behavioral therapy for insomnia improves sleep and decreases pain in older adults with co-morbid insomnia and osteoarthritis. J Clin Sleep Med 2009;5(4):355–62.
21. Manber R, Edinger JD, Gress JL, et al. Cognitive behavioral therapy for insomnia enhances depression outcome in patients with comorbid major depressive disorder and insomnia. Sleep 2008; 31(4):489–95.
22. Wilckens KA, Hall MH, Nebes RD, et al. Changes in cognitive performance are associated with changes in sleep in older adults with insomnia. Behav Sleep Med 2016;14(3):295–310.
23. Tyagi S, Resnick NM, Perera S, et al. Behavioral treatment of insomnia: also effective for nocturia. J Am Geriatr Soc 2014;62(1):54–60.
24. Germain A, Richardson R, Stocker R, et al. Treatment for insomnia in combat-exposed OEF/OIF/OND military veterans: preliminary randomized controlled trial. Behav Res Ther 2014;61:78–88.
25. Levenson JC, Rollman BL, Ritterband LM, et al. Hypertension with unsatisfactory sleep health (HUSH): study protocol for a randomized controlled trial. Trials 2017;18(1):256.
26. Foley D, Ancoli-Israel S, Britz P, et al. Sleep disturbances and chronic disease in older adults: results of the 2003 National Sleep Foundation Sleep in America Survey. J Psychosom Res 2004;56(5):497–502.
27. Glass J, Lanctot KL, Herrmann N, et al. Sedative hypnotics in older people with insomnia: meta-analysis of risks and benefits. BMJ 2005;331(7526):1169.
28. Bramoweth AD, Germain A, Youk AO, et al. A hybrid type I trial to increase Veterans' access to insomnia care: study protocol for a randomized controlled trial. Trials 2018;19(1):73.
29. McCrae CS, Bramoweth AD, Williams J, et al. Impact of brief cognitive behavioral treatment for insomnia on health care utilization and costs. J Clin Sleep Med 2014;10(2):127–35.
30. Koffel EA, Koffel JB, Gehrman PR. A meta-analysis of group cognitive behavioral therapy for insomnia. Sleep Med Rev 2015;19:6–16.
31. Morin CM. Insomnia. Psychological assessment and management. New York: Guilford Press; 1993.
32. Wohlgemuth WK, Edinger JD, Fins AI, et al. How many nights are enough? The short-term stability of sleep parameters in elderly insomniacs and normal sleepers. Psychophysiology 1999;36(2):233–44.
33. Chung KF, Lee CT, Yeung WF, et al. Sleep hygiene education as a treatment of insomnia: a systematic review and meta-analysis. Fam Pract 2018;35(4):365–75.
34. Borbely AA. A two process model of sleep regulation. Hum Neurobiol 1982;1(3):195–204.
35. Lack L, Wright H, Paynter D. The treatment of sleep onset insomnia with bright morning light. Sleep Biol Rhythms 2007;5(3):173–9.
36. Nau SD, McCrae CS, Cook KG, et al. Treatment of insomnia in older adults. Clin Psychol Rev 2005;25(5):645–72.
37. Spielman AJ, Caruso LS, Glovinsky PB. A behavioral-perspective on insomnia treatment. Psychiatr Clin North Am 1987;10(4):541–53.
38. Wang J, Wei Q, Wu X, et al. Brief behavioral treatment for patients with treatment-resistant insomnia. Neuropsychiatr Dis Treat 2016;12:1967–75.

Intensive Sleep Retraining Treatment of Insomnia

Leon Lack, PhD[a],*, Hannah Scott[a], Nicole Lovato, PhD[b]

KEYWORDS

- Insomnia • Sleep-onset insomnia • Intensive sleep retraining
- Cognitive and behavioral therapy for insomnia • Sleep deprivation
- Behavioral measure of sleep onset • Sleep-onset latency

KEY POINTS

- Multiple sleep-onset opportunities across the 24-hour day, allowing little sleep with each opportunity, show a dramatic reduction in sleep-onset latency in normal sleepers as well as those with insomnia.
- The use of multiple short sleep latencies during sleep deprivation forms the basis of a new behavioral treatment of insomnia, named intensive sleep retraining (ISR).
- ISR has been shown in 2 pilot studies and 1 randomized controlled trial to be an effective and durable treatment of insomnia.
- The original ISR studies were laboratory based and dependent on polysomnography (PSG) and PSG technician monitoring and, therefore, not readily available to the large insomnia population.
- The development of a behavioral measure of sleep onset with PSG accuracy has allowed the development of wearable and inexpensive devices to administer ISR in the home environment.

INTENSIVE SLEEP RETRAINING PROCEDURE

Intensive sleep retraining (ISR) was designed to be a behavioral treatment of insomnia. First, to understand its evolution, theoretic underpinnings, possible permutations, and treatment effectiveness, it is useful to describe its administration procedure. Patients attend the sleep laboratory approximately 2 hours before their typical bedtime and are set up for basic polysomnography (PSG) recording (electroencephalogram [EEG], electrooculogram, and electromyogram) simply for the detection of sleep onsets. It is advisable to instruct patients to restrict their sleep the previous night by approximately 2 hours to increase their homeostatic sleep drive for the laboratory session. Patients go to bed at their typical bedtime and attempt sleep while monitored by a trained sleep technician. The patient is allowed 25-minute opportunities in which to fall asleep every 30 minutes. If they do not initiate sleep during these opportunities, the trial is ended and they have a 5-minute time-out period before starting the next sleep opportunity trial. If they do initiate sleep (identified by 2–3 minutes of sustained sleep as judged by the technician) within a trial opportunity, they are awoken immediately for a wakeful time-out period before the next trial 30 minutes after the previous trial. Trials thus continue across the subsequent 24-hour period in the sleep laboratory, totaling 48 trials. At the completion of the trials, patients are allowed either to return home (driven by someone else) or remain in the laboratory to obtain a

Disclosure Statement: L. Lack is a shareholder in the company Re-Time Pty. Ltd. the manufacturer of the THIM device.
[a] College of Education, Psychology and Social Work, Flinders University, GPO Box 2100, Adelaide, SA 5001, Australia; [b] Adelaide Institute for Sleep Health, College of Medicine and Public Health, Flinders University, Mark Oliphant Building, GPO Box 2100, South Australia 5001, Australia
* Corresponding author.
E-mail address: leon.lack@flinders.edu.au

recovery sleep from their near 42 hours of effectively continuous wakefulness.

Because their brief episodes of light sleep during each sleep trial should not diminish their homeostatic sleep drive,[1] sleep pressure should remain high and continue to accumulate across the 24-hour laboratory period. In addition, a strong contribution from the circadian rhythm sleep phase across the 0100-hour to 0800-hour period[2,3] helps ensure rapid sleep onsets throughout the ISR procedure. Sleep-onset latency (SOL) is typically 15 minutes to 18 minutes in the first few trials but rapidly declines to less than 5 minutes from approximately 0300 hour onwards. During the course of the 24-hour procedure, patients typically experience more than 40 rapid SOLs less than 5 minutes in duration. Patients then usually experience a long and robust recovery sleep the following night and feel recovered from the sleep deprivation the following day. For convenience, the ISR procedure is usually carried out on a Friday or Saturday night so that patients can recover on the following Saturday or Sunday night, respectively. Although this procedure may seem tortuous (and patients have expressed some trepidation before entering the protocol), their experience is mainly one of heightened sleepiness, a somewhat reassuring feeling for patients who crave sleepiness but rarely experience it. None of the participants in the clinical trials withdrew participation despite the right to do so.

DEVELOPMENT HISTORICALLY

The seminal idea for ISR derived from basic circadian rhythm research in normal sleepers. The authors developed a modified methodology of the constant routine laboratory procedure[4] by including an ultradian sleep/wake schedule (10-minute sleep opportunities alternating with 20-minute wake periods) allowing circadian rhythm assessment of objective and subjective sleepiness in addition to the core body temperature rhythm.[3,5,6] These studies showed that during what is effectively total sleep deprivation combined with circadian rhythm effects, SOL dropped to very low levels (approximately 5 minutes) during the circadian night time and generally remained very low (<7 minutes) for the rest of the experimental laboratory procedure.

Gradisar and colleagues[7] tested differences in chronic insomnia patients compared with good sleepers in finger temperature changes at sleep onset. Both groups were involved in a 26-hour constant routine sleep deprivation procedure modified by the inclusion of half-hourly sleep latency trials, allowing for only 3 consecutive sleep epochs before being awoken. Despite having markedly longer subjective and objective SOLs in their home conditions, the insomnia group showed no differences in SOL compared with the good sleeper group across the 26-hour experimental procedure. At the beginning of the protocol in the late evening (9:00 PM–11:00 PM) both groups showed latencies of approximately 15 minutes, which rapidly dropped to approximately 8 minutes over the next 2 hours before decreasing further to approximately 5 minutes on average for both groups between 4:00 PM and 7:00 PM. SOLs then marginally increased over the course of the daytime period, reaching 10 minutes during the following evening for both groups (**Fig. 1**). This showed that the combination of homeostatic sleep drive from sleep deprivation plus high circadian sleep drive during the early/late morning

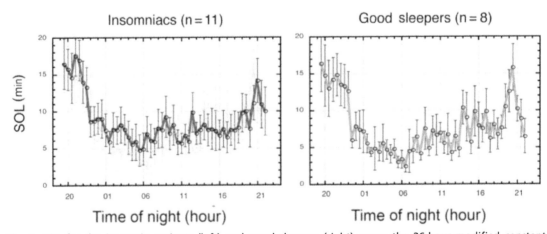

Fig. 1. SOL for the insomnia patients (left) and good sleepers (right) across the 26-hour modified constant routine, allowing half-hourly sleep-onset trials with participants awoken after only 3 consecutive 30-second epochs. (*From* Gradisar M, Lack L, Wright H, et al. Do chronic primary insomniacs have impaired heat loss when attempting sleep? Am J Physiol Regul Integr Comp Physiol 2006;290(4):R1118; with permission.)

maintained short SOLs in both groups of similar magnitude. This led to the realization that such a procedure may be therapeutic for patients with chronic sleep-onset insomnia.

FIRST CLINICAL TRIALS FOR THE TREATMENT OF INSOMNIA

The first pilot study was carried out in 2001 and reported at a conference the following year.[8] This short-term pilot study treated 10 chronic sleep-onset insomnia patients using ISR. Sleep was measured subjectively with sleep diaries and objectively with actigraphy for 2 weeks at baseline, 2 weeks immediately post-treatment, and 2 weeks at 8-week follow up. Sleep diary SOLs, on average, decreased from 75 minutes at baseline to 32 minutes post-treatment and to 45 minutes at follow-up, with both post-treatment latencies significantly less than at baseline. Total sleep time increased, on average, from 312 minutes to 397 minutes post-treatment and then to 372 minutes at follow-up, both significant improvements compared with baseline. Sleep efficiency improved 15% to 78%. Therefore, ISR was effective at treating chronic sleep-onset insomnia in this small sample.

These preliminary results were replicated in a further pilot study with a new group of 17 chronic sleep-onset insomnia patients.[9] The SOL data across the treatment protocol mirrored the earlier studies (**Fig. 2**). Improvements in sleep outcomes post-treatment also replicated the earlier pilot study, with SOL decreasing from 70 minutes to

39 minutes post-treatment and to 47 minutes at follow-up. Total sleep time also increased by 65 minutes at post-treatment and by 43 minutes at follow-up compared with baseline. Subsequently, sleep efficiency increased by 14% post-treatment and by 12% at follow-up compared with baseline.

These promising preliminary results of the clinical efficacy of ISR were sufficient to attract funding from the Australian National Health and Medical Research Council from 2004 to 2006 with Bootzin as coinvestigator. This allowed for a randomized controlled trial of the efficacy of ISR in comparison with stimulus control therapy (SCT),[10] which has been described as the "gold standard against which new interventions are tested."[11] SCT was the first behavioral treatment specifically for insomnia and remains the most effective single-component treatment. One arm of the randomized controlled trial combined ISR with SCT, where patients underwent ISR on 1 night and then SCT over the next 4 weeks. All treatment arms were compared with a waitlist control group, whereby 80 patients with sleep-onset insomnia were randomly allocated to the 4 groups. The results of this study were published in the premier journal, *Sleep*,[12] and also selected for editorial comment in that issue.[13] The 2 Harris and colleagues[9,12] studies have both received 27 citations and continue to be cited at a consistent rate.

Harris and colleagues[12] again showed the consistent shortening of SOL across the ISR protocol (**Fig. 3**). Of most interest, however, were the sustained effects on sleep outcomes at

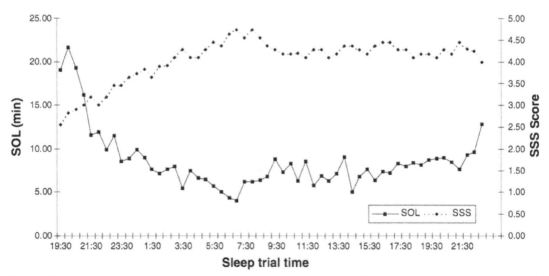

Fig. 2. SOL means and subjective sleepiness (Stanford Sleepiness Scale [SSS] Score) means across the 26-hour ISR treatment period. (*From* Harris J, Lack L, Wright H, et al. Intensive sleep retraining treatment for chronic primary insomnia: a preliminary investigation. J Sleep Res 2007;16(3):279; with permission.)

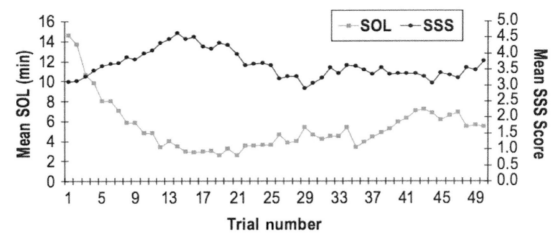

Fig. 3. Mean SOL and Stanford Sleepiness Scale (SSS) score by trial number during the ISR treatment procedure. (*From* Harris J, Lack L, Kemp K, et al. A randomized controlled trial of intensive sleep retraining (ISR): a brief conditioning treatment for chronic insomnia. Sleep 2012;35(1):54; with permission.)

post-treatment and long-term follow-up. ISR alone was as effective as SCT in reducing SOL and increasing total sleep time and sleep efficiency at post-treatment (after 4 weeks of SCT) and at 2-months' and 6-months' follow-up. The improvements for the ISR treatment emerged immediately after the 24-hour treatment protocol compared with the same degree of change after 4 weeks of SCT. The instructions for SCT involve getting out of bed if not asleep within 15 minutes of lights out until finally a short (<15-minute) sleep onset occurs. Thus, SCT ensures 1 rapid sleep onset on each night of therapy. The ISR procedure, on the other hand, guarantees a large number of rapid sleep onsets (typically >40 sleep onsets) over the course of one 24-hour period. Essentially, it compresses the experience of 5 weeks of SCT into 1 day. This is the most parsimonious explanation for the benefits of ISR in comparison with SCT.

A combination of ISR and SCT over the following 4 weeks provided generally greater improvements in sleep and daytime functioning measures than either treatment alone. Results from the combined condition showed the rapidity of response similar to the ISR condition but with the added benefit of greater sustained improvements at follow-up, presumably provided by the 4 weeks of SCT. In this condition, ISR essentially provided a therapeutic kickstart with the continued instructions of SCT maintaining and extending the gains in the long term. One of the allures of pharmacotherapy for insomnia treatment is the rapidity of improvement within the first night or first week of administration. The rapidity of treatment response from ISR may provide an allure to compete with pharmacotherapy that current behavioral therapies, taking 3 weeks to 6 weeks to be effective, do not have.

With its strong and rapid effect, ISR could become the treatment of choice for patients and physicians for the treatment of insomnia.

Translating intensive sleep retraining beyond the sleep laboratory

Although ISR is an effective treatment of insomnia, the laboratory-based procedure as described is not a practical implementation method. ISR requires patients to undergo overnight PSG recording with a sleep technician monitoring PSG in real time to detect sleep onset and to wake the patient up after 2 minutes to 3 minutes of light sleep during each trial. This laboratory-based procedure is costly, limited in opportunity, and simply not available to most insomnia patients. Therefore, until a practical alternative administration method is developed, the therapeutic benefits of ISR cannot be realized on a large scale. To quote the late Arthur Spielman, the developer of another major behavioral therapy for insomnia known as bedtime restriction[14]:

The findings of Harris and colleagues (2012) suggest that ISR approach holds great promise. Patients await a non-drug treatment for insomnia that brings relief as rapidly as medication. Clinicians in the community look forward to more widely applicable ISR-like procedures that can be implemented at home, without expensive and complicated sleep technology, by non-sleep experts. Theoreticians anticipate tests of the learning, sleep perception, and cognitive explanations of ISR's rapid and robust benefits. This stunning demonstration by Harris and colleagues should serve as a challenge to the field to create the next generation of theoretically driven non-pharmacological treatments for insomnia.[13]

Recognizing this challenge, sleep technologist and clinical sleep educator Michael Schwartz developed the Sleep On Cue smartphone application (app) to translate the ISR protocol to the home environment.[15] To undergo ISR, a user lies down in bed while holding a smartphone and wearing earphones and attempts to fall asleep. The app emits a faint tone stimulus via the earphones approximately every 30 seconds and the user is required to move the smartphone in response. When the user fails to respond to the tone stimulus, the app assumes that the user has fallen asleep and emits a strong vibration to awake the user. Research with the iPhone app and similar devices have shown this an accurate method of estimating sleep onset, with responses tending to cease 2 minutes to 3 minutes after the onset of EEG N1 sleep.[16–19] Therefore, Sleep On Cue app users are likely to experience the desired 2 minutes to 3 minutes of light sleep before they are woken up, aligning with the laboratory-based administration method. After the strong vibration has woken the user, there is a short break before initiating the next trial, and this cycle continues overnight until the following morning. The next day, users can view their SOLs on the Sleep On Cue app, providing feedback about how rapidly they were able to fall asleep. Because the administration of the ISR protocol is similar to the laboratory-based method, the Sleep On Cue app should be successful in carrying out the ISR procedure in a patient's home without the need for PSG or sleep technicians.

The app developers have reported considerable anecdotal support from their customers, but experimental confirmation of treatment efficacy is still preliminary.[20] This pilot study compared sleep outcome measures at baseline to post-treatment and 4-week follow-up in 12 drug-free chronic insomnia patients. The study also tested a modified ISR protocol whereby sleep-onset trials were separated by only a brief 6-minute break compared with 1 sleep-onset trial every 30 minutes. Using this modified ISR protocol, participants completed more than 30 trials within a 10-hour nighttime period. Patients then stayed awake across the following day and allowed themselves a 9-hour sleep opportunity for their recovery sleep the following night. This study showed improvements in sleep and daytime functioning measures comparable to those of the earlier pilot studies.[8,9] Therefore, it seems that ISR can be administered in the home environment with good adherence without experimenter supervision, and treatment

effectiveness is at least comparable to the earlier laboratory-based administration method.

Although Sleep On Cue has the capacity to administer the ISR protocol, there are issues pertaining to the user experience of the app. The use of tone stimulus is problematic because the external stimulus should be maintained at the lowest perceptible intensity across the treatment protocol to minimize the disruption of the stimulus on the process of falling asleep while remaining perceptible to users so they can initiate the required behavioral response. Maintaining this intensity using a tone stimulus emitted via earphones is difficult, because they may become dislodged overnight. Perhaps most problematic is the requirement that users hold their smartphone while undergoing the ISR procedure. Users are required to move their phone with a back-and-forth motion of the wrist in response to the tone stimuli. The effort and motor movement required to produce this response may contribute to unnecessarily prolonged wakefulness during the ISR protocol. Many individuals also do not like having their smartphone in the bedroom environment while they are attempting sleep. Overcoming these issues may create a more user-friendly experience and greater treatment adherence and satisfaction.

In collaboration with Re-Time, the authors developed a small ring-like device (THIM, Re-Time Pty Ltd, China) to administer ISR in the home environment.[21] Users attempt to fall asleep while wearing THIM on the index finger. The device emits a low-intensity, short-duration vibration approximately every 30 seconds to which users respond with a gentle finger twitch. If THIM detects a response to the vibration, the device assumes the user is awake, and, when they cease responding, THIM assumes they have fallen asleep. This is a similar method of estimating sleep onset as Sleep On Cue, except that THIM uses tactile rather than auditory stimuli, removing the need for uncomfortable earphones. The device also uses finger twitches for the required behavioral response rather than more onerous hand motions, which likely are less cumbersome and bothersome for the user. Once THIM detects sleep onset, it emits an intense vibration to wake the user. After a short break, the user can attempt another sleep-onset trial. The THIM-administered ISR protocol aligns with the laboratory-based ISR protocol, with the user falling asleep and waking up shortly thereafter on many occasions during the treatment session. The device is programmable using a smartphone but then administers the ISR protocol independently, meaning that users do not need to have their smartphone in the bedroom environment.

Similar to uses of behavioral response measures of PSG-defined sleep onset, discussed previously, THIM determination of behavioral sleep onset is also a valid measure of PSG sleep onset.[22]

THIM is also a sleep tracker using the well-established and well-utilized actigraphy method of measuring sleep overnight.[23] Using the device's built-in accelerometer, if THIM detects a significant amount of movement, then the user must be awake, and, if there is little or no movement, the user is likely asleep. Unlike other consumer sleep trackers that track only sleep and unlike Sleep On Cue that only administers ISR to treat insomnia, THIM is capable of both tracking and treating sleep. This dual capability means that THIM may be more useful for consumers wanting to monitor and treat their poor sleep. Therefore, the development of smartphone apps to administer ISR has met the first stated hope of Spielman and Glovinsky,[13] that ISR can be translated from the bench to the bedside[24] and be readily available to the large insomnia suffering public. The authors currently are assessing the efficacy of THIM-administered ISR for treating insomnia in a pilot case-control study. The comprehensive assessment of the effectiveness of this home administered ISR using either Sleep On Cue or THIM applications awaits robust randomized controlled trials.

WHERE TO FROM HERE?

The development of a practical method of administering ISR outside the sleep laboratory has opened the doors for more research to improve the ISR treatment protocol. Testing the individual components of the ISR treatment will address the aspiration of Spielman and Glovinsky[13] for a deeper understanding of the components that lead to the greatest therapeutic benefit. A greater theoretic understanding of ISR will help refine the treatment procedure to maximize its effectiveness and adherence.

Learning theory suggests the main effective components of the ISR protocol are the numerous trials with rapid sleep onsets. Each of these trials reassociates going to bed, turning out the lights, assuming a comfortable sleeping position, and intending to fall asleep with a rapid sleep-onset experience rather than persistent wakefulness. The rapidity of the sleep onset obviates any anxieties or frustrations normally experienced with prolonged sleep latencies. From an operant conditioning perspective, the stimuli and circumstances surrounding the sleep attempts would develop greater stimulus control to produce the sleep-onset response. From a classical conditioning perspective, the conditioned response in chronic insomnia of anxiety and frustration (sympathetic nervous system response of fight or flight) elicited by the stimuli surrounding the attempt to fall asleep would gradually extinguish and allow the biological determinants of sleep (high homeostatic drive and circadian sleep phase) to trigger sleep without interference.

Assuming that learning is an important component of ISR, there are several questions about the number of and administration protocol for the sleep-onset trials to produce the greatest improvements. For example, how many trials would be necessary on average to produce a clinically meaningful response? The authors expect a nonlinear relationship between number of trials and sleep improvement, with the initial rapid sleep-onset experiences providing more increment of benefit than latter trials, a negative exponential function or law of diminishing returns. This may be a practical consideration because insisting on a large number of trials (eg, > 40 trials) is likely to be more arduous and less likely to gain treatment adherence. For example, if 20 rapid sleep-onset trials gained 90% of the benefit of 40 trials but took half as long to complete and subsequently led to much less sleep deprivation and greater treatment adherence, then that should be the recommended ISR administration protocol.

If patients purchase an app or wearable device to administer ISR, then the treatment will be available for more than 1 application at home as opposed to the original laboratory-based administration, which is practically restricted by cost to a single extended laboratory session. Consequently, users could complete ISR for a few hours over multiple nights rather than a marathon session in 1 night. If this is equally effective to a single extended retraining session, it may be preferred in practice and receive greater treatment adherence and presumably greater treatment benefit. Because distributed practice trials are more efficient than massed practice,[25] and if this phenomenon is applicable for learning rapid sleep onsets, then the authors would recommend distributing sleep-onset trials over multiple nights. This speculation, however, needs to be tested experimentally.

Changing the original application from a single treatment session to several shorter sessions may have an unanticipated negative impact if it affected other possible therapeutic elements of ISR. Such a potential therapeutic component of ISR could be the experience of total sleep deprivation that is inherent in a single long session. Patients with chronic insomnia typically believe in the negative effects of sleep loss more strongly than good sleepers.[26] As discussed previously, a common anecdotal report is trepidation at the thought of undergoing sleep deprivation in the ISR protocol. Although patients may need some encouragement to do so, their experience of sleep deprivation may actually be therapeutic. The subjective experience of the laboratory-based ISR protocol was increasingly strong feelings of sleepiness.[12] As discussed previously, these feelings are not aversive to those with chronic insomnia who typically feel fatigue rather than sleepiness.[27] Feelings of sleepiness may be reassuring to patients because they are a sign of the sought-after increased sleep propensity. Furthermore, the experience of total sleep deprivation without aversive consequences may help disconfirm their belief that sleep loss per se will lead to severe daytime impairments and aversive feelings. In other words, the experience would inoculate patients against their typical anxiety of sleep loss and be an effective cognitive therapy instrument.[28] This would reduce the strength of the maladaptive belief that helps fuel and perpetuate the insomnia.

Another possible cognitive element of chronic insomnia addressed by ISR is the anxiety that patients have lost the ability to sleep or that their sleep mechanism has in some way become permanently damaged, leading to a lifetime of insomnia suffering.[26] Anecdotal evidence from the previous ISR clinical studies is that after the approximately 40 hours of sleep loss experienced in the ISR protocol, patients typically experienced a robust recovery sleep that was longer with higher sleep efficiency than they had experienced for a long time and felt much better than usual the following day. This demonstrated to them that their sleep mechanism responds normally to sleep loss and was not irreparably damaged. Although this anecdotal evidence needs to be investigated further, earlier studies have shown a normal recovery sleep after sleep deprivation in insomnia sufferers.[29]

Furthermore, this 1 relatively benign experience of extreme sleep deprivation could make adjunct add-on behavioral therapies, such as SCT or bedtime restriction therapy, more likely to receive adherence. Both these therapies involve mild sleep loss and may normally suffer compliance problems because of the fear of sleep loss. After the easy survival of total sleep loss, however, the degree of mild sleep loss in these adjunct behavioral therapies would seem much less threatening and, thus, be more likely to receive adherence.

Additionally, ISR may address the misperceptions of sleep loss and time taken to initially fall asleep, both typically overestimated by insomnia patients.[30] During the ISR procedure administered in the laboratory and by the Sleep On Cue app and THIM device at home, feedback is given of actual time taken to fall asleep after each sleep-onset trial. This may help correct the sleep misperception typical with insomnia[31] and increase the perceived total sleep time obtained each night. This would also reduce the discrepancy between estimated total sleep and the amount of sleep patients believe they need thus reducing the anxiety about the degree of harm their sleep may be producing. This overestimated sleep loss has also been identified as one of the cognitive elements tending to exacerbate insomnia.[28]

The extent to which these 3 possible cognitive therapy elements (total sleep deprivation, robust recovery sleep, and corrected sleep perception) contributes to the effectiveness of ISR needs to be investigated to determine the most effective and efficient administration in the home environment. In the extreme case that sleep deprivation and robust recovery sleep account for the large majority of the benefits of ISR, a more practical treatment could dispense with the numerous sleep-onset trials and simply use total sleep deprivation across 1 night as the therapy. If, at on the other extreme, the sleep deprivation and recovery sleep elements account for little of the therapeutic benefit, then the ISR protocol may be more efficiently administered over multiple nights with only 2 hours to 3 hours of sleep retraining per night, thus avoiding total sleep deprivation and its detrimental effects across the following day. If all these components, discussed previously, contribute significantly on average to the effectiveness of ISR, then, armed with this knowledge, patients may opt for the procedure most practical for them, which most likely leads to the greatest treatment adherence.

An increasing focus of insomnia research is phenotyping insomnia to investigate the most appropriate and thus most effective elements of cognitive behavioral therapy.[32,33] Further investigations may be directed at phenotyping different types of insomnia that may respond more effectively to 1 element of ISR rather than another. These are all questions begging to be investigated and worth investigating given the high effectiveness of ISR. In the words of Spielman and Glovinsky,[13] this research will help, "to create the next generation of theoretically driven non-pharmacological treatments for insomnia." Furthermore, with the invention of practical ISR administration methods, this effective treatment can be translated to the home environment and available to treat insomnia on a large scale.

REFERENCES

1. Tietzel AJ, Lack LC. The recuperative value of brief and ultra-brief naps on alertness and cognitive performance. J Sleep Res 2002;11(3):213–8.

2. Dijk D-J, Czeisler CA. Paradoxical timing of the circadian rhythm of sleep propensity serves to consolidate sleep and wakefulness in humans. Neurosci Lett 1994;166(1):63–8.

3. Lack L, Lushington K. The rhythms of human sleep propensity and core body temperature. J Sleep Res 1996;5(1):1–11.

4. Czeisler C, Brown E, Ronda J, et al. A clinical method to assess the endogenous circadian phase (ECP) of the deep circadian oscillator in man. Sleep Res 1985;14:295.

5. Gradisar M, Lack L. Relationships between the circadian rhythms of finger temperature, core temperature, sleep latency, and subjective sleepiness. J Biol Rhythms 2004;19(2):157–63.

6. Lack L, Gradisar M. Acute finger temperature changes preceding sleep onset over a 45-h period. J Sleep Res 2002;11(4):275–82.

7. Gradisar M, Lack L, Wright H, et al. Do chronic primary insomniacs have impaired heat loss when attempting sleep? Am J Physiol Regul Integr Comp Physiol 2006;290(4):R1115–21.

8. Lack L, Baraniec M. Intensive sleep onset training for sleep onset insomnia. Sleep 2002;25(Abstract Supplement):A478–9.

9. Harris J, Lack L, Wright H, et al. Intensive sleep retraining treatment for chronic primary insomnia: a preliminary investigation. J Sleep Res 2007;16(3):276–84.

10. Bootzin RR. Stimulus control treatment for insomnia. Proc Am Psychol Assoc 1972;7:395–6.

11. Bootzin R, Epstein DR. Understanding and treating insomnia. Annu Rev Clin Psychol 2011;7:435–58.

12. Harris J, Lack L, Kemp K, et al. A randomized controlled trial of intensive sleep retraining (ISR): a brief conditioning treatment for chronic insomnia. Sleep 2012;35(1):49–60.

13. Spielman AJ, Glovinsky PB. What a difference a day makes. Sleep 2012;35(1):11–2.

14. Spielman AJ, Saskin P, Thorpy MJ. Treatment of chronic insomnia by restriction of time in bed. Sleep 1987;10:45–56.

15. MicroSleep. Sleep on cue-research application (version 1.1) 2015. https://itunes.apple.com/au/app/sleep-on-cue/id829583727?mt=8. Accessed April 18, 2017.

16. Connelly L. Behavioural measurements of sleep onset: a comparison of two devices [Honours thesis]. Adelaide (Australia): Flinders University; 2004.

17. The relationship between EEG and a behavioural measure of sleep onset. 1995. Available at: http://hdl.handle.net/2328/36963. Accessed January 08, 2019.

18. Scott H, Lack L. The revival of active behavioural devices for measuring sleep latency. SM Journal of Sleep Disorders 2017;3(2):1015.

19. Ogilvie RD, Wilkinson RT, Allison S. The detection of sleep onset: behavioral, physiological, and subjective convergence. Sleep 1989;12(5):458–74.

20. Mair A, Lack L, Scott H. Mobile phone technology to administer an effective behaviour therapy for insomnia in patient's homes. J Sleep Res 2018;27(Abstract Supplement):12–3.

21. Re-Time. Thim - the first wearable device for sleep, which will improve your sleep. 2016. Available at: http://thim.io/. Accessed February 01, 2019.

22. Scott H, Lack L, Lovato N. The validity of a novel wearable device for estimating sleep onset. J Sleep Res 2018;27(Abstract Supplement):30.

23. Smith MT, McCrae CS, Cheung J, et al. Use of actigraphy for the evaluation of sleep disorders and circadian rhythm sleep-wake disorders: an american academy of sleep medicine systematic review, meta-analysis, and GRADE assessment. J Clin Sleep Med 2018;14(7):1209–30.

24. Lack L, Scott H, Micic G, et al. Intensive sleep retraining: from bench to bedside. Brain Sci 2017;7(4) [pii:E33].

25. Baddeley AD, Longman DJA. The influence of length and frequency of training sessions on the rate of learning to type. Ergonomics 1978;21(8):627–35.

26. Morin CM, Stone J, Trinkle D, et al. Dysfunctional beliefs and attitudes about sleep among older adults with and without insomnia complaints. Psychol Aging 1993;8(3):463–7.

27. Gradisar M, Lack L, Richards H, et al. The flinders fatigue scale: preliminary psychometric properties and clinical sensitivity of a new scale for measuring daytime fatigue associated with insomnia. J Clin Sleep Med 2007;3(7):722–8.

28. Harvey AG. A cognitive theory and therapy for chronic insomnia. J Cogn Psychother 2005;19(1):41–59.

29. Bonnet MH. Effect of 64hours of sleep deprivation upon sleep in geriatric normal and insomniacs. Neurobiol Aging 1986;7(2):89–96.

30. Carskadon MA, Dement WC, Mitler MM, et al. Self-reports versus sleep laboratory findings in 122 drug-free subjects with complaints of chronic insomnia. Am J Psychiatry 1976;133(12):1382–8.

31. Mercer JD, Bootzin RR, Lack LC. Insomniacs' perception of wake instead of sleep. Sleep 2002;25(5):564–71.

32. Bathgate CJ, Edinger JD, Krystal AD. Insomnia patients with objective short sleep duration have a blunted response to cognitive behavioural therapy for insomnia. Sleep 2017;40(1):zsw012.

33. Lovato N, Lack L, Kennaway DJ. Comparing and contrasting therapeutic effects of cognitive-behaviour therapy for older adults suffering from insomnia with short and long objective sleep duration. Sleep Med 2016;22:4–12.

Cognitive Behavioral Therapies for Insomnia and Hypnotic Medications
Considerations and Controversies

Janet M.Y. Cheung, PhD[a,b,c], Xiao-Wen Ji, PhD[b,c],
Charles M. Morin, PhD[b,c],*

KEYWORDS

- Cognitive behavioral therapy for insomnia • Pharmacotherapy • Stepped care
- Treatment preference • Combination therapy • Treatment sequencing

KEY POINTS

- Insomnia is a prevalent and costly health problem that often remains untreated or is treated inadequately. There are, however, several evidence-based treatment options, including cognitive behavioral therapies (CBTs) and pharmacologic therapies, each with its own advantages and limitations.
- Medications with specific indications for insomnia produce rapid symptomatic relief, but there is little to no evidence that sleep improvements are maintained after drug discontinuation or long-term, continued usage. Conversely, CBT takes longer than drugs to produce sleep improvements, but these improvements are well sustained over time.
- Aside from their short-term and long-term benefits, other key considerations need to be taken into account when selecting among the different insomnia therapies. These include patients' treatment preferences, how best to deliver CBT, whether to combine or sequence CBTs and medication therapies, and who should treat insomnia. These considerations may have a significant impact on efficacy, compliance, attrition, and access to treatment.
- Several innovative treatment delivery methods relying on digital technology are increasingly used to treat insomnia. Although these self-help approaches may reduce cost and human resources and increase access, an important shortcoming is the high attrition rate during the course of these self-guided approaches.
- The publications of clinical practice guidelines by several international medical and sleep organizations have reached the same recommendation, that is, CBT should be the first-line treatment of insomnia, and only when such treatment is not available or not effective should medication be considered for treating persistent insomnia. It is hoped that such strong and uniform endorsement by the medical and sleep community will help narrow the current gap between the available research evidence and clinical practices.

[a] School of Pharmacy, Faculty of Medicine and Health, The University of Sydney, Room S303, Pharmacy and Bank Building (A15), Science Road, Camperdown Campus, Sydney, NSW 2006, Australia; [b] École de psychologie, Université Laval, Pavillon Félix-Antoine-Savard, local 1036, Québec, QC G1V 0A6, Canada; [c] Centre d'étude des troubles du sommeil, Institut universitaire en santé mentale de Québec, Québec, QC, Canada
* Corresponding author. Pavillon Félix-Antoine-Savard, local 1030 2325, rue des Bibliothèques, Québec, QC G1V 0A6, Canada.
E-mail address: cmorin@psy.ulaval.ca

Sleep Med Clin 14 (2019) 253–265
https://doi.org/10.1016/j.jsmc.2019.01.006
1556-407X/19/© 2019 Elsevier Inc. All rights reserved.

INTRODUCTION

Insomnia is a highly prevalent condition with consequences on next-day functioning (eg, fatigue, reduced energy, poor attention, and mood disturbances) as well as long-term negative outcomes on physical (eg, hypertension), mental (eg, depression), and occupational (eg, reduced productivity) health. Despite, these negative impacts, few people with insomnia seek treatment and even fewer receive adequate treatment. Nevertheless, there are several treatment options available for the management of insomnia and these can be broadly defined into 3 classes—pharmacologic, cognitive behavioral, and complementary and alternative therapies; and, each of these can be further divided into several subclasses. The levels of evidence supporting these therapies vary significantly, as do the potential adverse events. Although the discourse around the optimal treatment of insomnia has centered on the divide between the use or nonuse of medications, there are several other key considerations when selecting a treatment of the management of insomnia. This article reviews some of these key considerations and controversies. After summarizing the evidence derived from meta-analyses on the efficacy of the 3 main treatment options, other critical issues are addressed, such as whether medication should be used at all in treating insomnia and, if so, how best to combine or sequence different treatment modalities, what to do with treatment-resistant patients, treatment preferences and compliance, who should be treating insomnia, and optimal methods of treatment delivery. This article concludes with an appraisal of what the future might hold with the recent advent of clinical practice guidelines for treating insomnia and some recommendations for future research.

EVIDENCE FOR EFFICACY—COGNITIVE BEHAVIORAL THERAPY FOR INSOMNIA AND MEDICATION USED SINGLY AND IN COMBINATION
Evidence for Pharmacotherapy

Until recently, benzodiazepines (BZDs) and non-BZD receptor agonists (Z-drugs), working via the γ-aminobutyric acid (GABA) pathway, have been the mainstay of pharmacotherapy for insomnia. Newer agents for insomnia include the melatonin receptor agonist ramelteon, low-dose doxepin (3–6 mg), and the orexin receptor antagonist suvorexant. Owing to the short duration of clinical drug trials, there is currently insufficient evidence on the long-term efficacy of pharmacologic agents. Current guidelines recommend only short-term use of these agents (<4 weeks) where nonpharmacologic options are not preferred or unavailable.[1,2] The general adverse effects profile of pharmacotherapy, such as residual sedation, memory loss, tolerance, and dependence, also limits their use long term.[3,4]

In a meta-analysis of 31 studies of randomized controlled drug trials (n = 3820; trial duration range 2–224 days) of BZDs, Z-drugs, and antidepressants, significant improvements were observed across a range of objective sleep measures captured by polysomnography. Pooled effect size (ES) (95% CI) at post-treatment for sleep-onset latency (SOL) was −0.36 (−0.44, −0.27) and wake time after sleep onset (WASO) was −0.29 (−0.36, −0.23) and total sleep time (TST) was 0.27 (0.17, 0.38). Post-treatment sleep efficiency (SE) also improved, with a small ES of 0.29 (0.21, 0.37). At the therapeutic class level, the largest effects were observed for BZDs followed by Z-drugs and antidepressants.[5] **Fig. 1**A summarizes the ESs of the respective outcomes captured by polysomnography and self-reported sleep diaries.

For ramelteon, a meta-analysis of 13 studies (n = 5812; treatment duration range 6–180 days) showed, based on weighted mean differences (95% CI), a reduction of SOL by 9.36 minutes (−12.35, −6.36), no change for WASO, an increase in TST by 7.26 minutes (2.47, 12.06), and an improvement in SE by 4.42% (0.42, 8.42). Only a small effect at post-treatment (treatment duration range 6–180 days), however, was observed for sleep quality −0.07 (−013, −0.02).[4] A recently published meta-analysis of 4 studies (n = 3076; treatment duration range 4–52 weeks) on suvorexant at doses ranging from 15 mg to 40 mg showed improved sleep quality, with a small ES (95% CI) of 0.33 (0.21, 0.46), with effects sustained at 3-month and 12-month follow-ups. Based on weighted mean differences (95% CI), SOL was reduced by 10.79 minutes (−13.99, −7.60), WASO was reduced by 25.86 minutes (−30.19, −21.53), and subjective TST increased by 20.10 minutes (14.19, 26.00). Measures of SE were not included in the analyses but improvement in subjective sleep quality was maintained at 12 months, with an ES of 0.20 (0.01–0.40).[6]

Although discussion of prescribing practices is beyond the scope of this article, the current position of the American Academy of Sleep Medicine (AASM) does not recommend off-label use of antipsychotics, antiepileptics, or antidepressants.[1,2,7] A recent Cochrane review investigating the efficacy, safety, and tolerability of antidepressants used for adults with insomnia converges with AASM recommendations. Specifically, the pooled

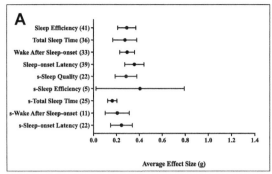 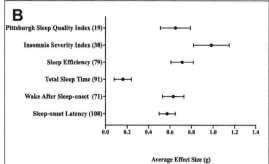

Fig. 1. Average ESs of the efficacy of treatments of insomnia. (*A*) Shows the pooled ESs of pharmacotherapy (ie, BZDs, Z-drugs, and low-dose doxepin) for insomnia across sleep measures captured by polysomnography and sleep diary adapted using data from Winkler and colleagues. (*B*) Shows the pooled ESs of CBT-I based on sleep diary and clinical measures adapted using data from van Straten and colleagues. s-, subjective sleep parameters (derived from sleep diary). (*Data from* [*A*] Winkler A, Auer C, Doering BK, et al. Drug treatment of primary insomnia: a meta-analysis of polysomnographic randomized controlled trials. CNS Drugs 2014;28(9):799–816; and [*B*] van Straten A, van der Zweerde T, Kleiboer A, et al. Cognitive and behavioral therapies in the treatment of insomnia: a meta-analysis. Sleep Med Rev 2018;38:3–16.)

mean difference from 4 studies on doxepin compared with placebo (n = 518 participants) showed no impact on SOL but WASO was reduced by 14.63 minutes (−25.99, −3.27), TST increased by 22.88 minutes (13.17, 32.59), and SE improved by 6.29% (3.17, 9.41). A moderate improvement in subjective sleep quality was also observed (−0.39 [−0.56, −0.21]). The meta-analyses for the 3 studies comparing trazodone to placebo (n = 370) showed moderate improvements in subjective sleep outcomes −0.34 (−0.66, −0.02) but little to no effect on SE (1.38% [−2.87, 5.63]).[8] Despite short-term improvements in sleep quality, there is still a need for high-quality trials on antidepressant use in insomnia and better reporting of adverse effects (ie, residual sedation and dry mouth) to make conclusive recommendations.

Treatment guidelines similarly recommend against the use of over-the-counter sleep aids (eg, diphenhydramine and doxylamine) and herbal remedies/dietary supplements despite their widespread use among consumers.[1,2,7] A recent systematic review on herbal medicines (n = 1602), including valerian, kava, chamomile, and wuling, concluded that there was insufficient evidence for using these agents in the management of insomnia.[9] Specifically, valerian did not significantly improve SOL, sleep duration, SE, or subjective sleep quality in the meta-analyses conducted as part of the systematic review.

In summary, sedative-hypnotic medications, at least those with a specific indication for insomnia, may be clinically useful for short-term or situational insomnia. Although this recommendation for short-term use is disconnected from the clinical profile of many patients who experience chronic insomnia, there is little evidence of sustained efficacy with

prolonged medication usage and no evidence of sustained sleep improvement after its discontinuation.

Evidence for Cognitive Behavioral Therapy for Insomnia

Table 1 provides an overview of recent meta-analyses on the efficacy of CBT for insomnia (CBT-I) delivered according to different formats (individual, group, and Internet based). Findings from these meta-analyses provide strong evidence that multicomponent CBT-I has a positive impact on several symptoms of insomnia disorder presenting with or without comorbid conditions. In a meta-analysis of 11 studies (n = 1460) on Internet-based CBT-I, the pooled ES (95% CI) at post-treatment was 0.41 (0.29, 0.53) for SOL, 0.45 (0.25, 0.66) for WASO, 0.29 (0.17, 0.42) for TST, and 0.58 (0.36, 0.81) for SE.[10] Compared with digital CBT-I (dCBT-I), the pooled ESs from 5 studies (n = 608) were greater for group CBT-I across SOL (0.77 [0.54, 0.99]), WASO (0.89 [0.60, 1.17]), and SE (1.13 [0.70, 1.56]).[11] Comparable ESs were observed, however, for TST (0.29 [0.11, 0.46]). In another meta-analysis that reported similar outcomes, some of the largest ESs were obtained on patient-reported outcomes, such as the Insomnia Severity Index (ES 0.98) and the Pittsburgh Sleep Quality Index (PSQI) (ES 0.65), as highlighted in **Fig. 1**B.[12]

Furthermore, the presence of psychiatric comorbidities did not seem to alter the treatment effects of CBT-I. For the respective sleep parameters, the moderate to large ESs observed were similar to those typically reported for patients without comorbid psychiatric or medical disorders.[13–15] Only 2

Table 1
Summary of recent meta-analyses on cognitive behavioral therapies for insomnia and the management of insomnia

	Treatment Format	Specific Program Features	Improvement in Sleep-onset Sleep-onset Latency, Post-treatment	Improvement in Wake After Sleep Onset, Post-treatment	Improvement in Total Sleep Time, Post-treatment	Improvement in Sleep Efficiency, Post-treatment	Subjective Sleep Quality, Post-treatment	Notes
Brasure et al,[16] 2016	Psychological and behavioral interventions for insomnia (at least 4 wk of treatment)	Only present multi-component CBT-I in varied delivery modes	Favors CBT-I WMD −11.63 (−16.55, −6.71) minutes	Favors CBT-I WMD −21.39 (−35.78, −7.00) minutes	Not significant WMD 11.00 (−0.06, −22.05) minutes	Favors CBT-I WMD 6.86 (4.55, −9.16) %	ISI: WMD −4.78 (−6.45 to −3.11) PSQI: WMD −2.10 (−2.87 to −1.34); n = 6	n = 20 (total study number is 61); compare CBT-I with an inactive control group
Geiger-Brown et al,[17] 2015	Face-to-face, multicomponent CBT-I (individual or group)	Must include stimulus control and sleep restriction	WMD 20.68 (SE 3.27)	WMD 20.79 (SE 3.60)	WMD 17.09 (SE 5.16)	WMD 9.25 (SE 1.24)	ISI: WMD 6.36 (SE 1.27) PSQI: WMD 3.30 (SE 0.44)	23 studies, including 1379 patients with medical and psychiatric diagnoses
Ho et al,[13] 2016	CBT-I or/and CBT-based IRT	For sleep disturbances in patients with PTSD (individual or group)	ES −0.83 (95% CI, −1.19, −0.47), N = 4	ES −1.02 (95% CI, −1.39, −0.66), N = 4	ES 0.39 (95% CI, −0.05, 0.84) not significant N = 4	ES 1.15 (95% CI, 0.75, 1.56), N = 5	ISI: ES −1.15, (95% CI, −1.81, −0.49) N = 5 PSQI: ES −0.87, (95% CI, −1.18, −0.56) N = 6	11 trials of 593 participants; between-ES, compared with WL/ psychoeducation (standardized mean difference)

Study	Intervention	Population						Notes
Johnson et al,[14] 2016	CBT-I (in variations)	For cancer survivors	ES 0.43 (95% CI, 0.27, 0.58)	ES 0.41 (95% CI, 0.24, 0.59)	ES 0.53 (95% CI, 0.39, 0.68)	ISI: ES 0.77(95% CI, 0.60; 0.93)		8 trials of total 752 cancer survivors; ES from preintervention to postintervention compared with control group ES: Cohen's d
Koffel et al,[11] 2015	CBT-I was delivered in a group format of 2 or more patients	Include both behavioral and cognitive treatment	ES 0.77 (95% CI, 0.54, 0.99)	ES 0.89 (95% CI, 0.60, 1.17)	ES 0.29 (95% CI, 0.11, 0.46)	ES 1.13 (95% CI, 0.70, 1.56)	Subjective sleep quality ES 0.85 (95% CI, 0.57.1.14)	5 studies of 608 participants ES: Hedge's g
Trauer et al,[18] 2015	Face-to-face CBT-I	Incorporated at least 3 of the following: cognitive therapy, stimulus control, sleep restriction, sleep hygiene, and relaxation	19.03 (95% CI, 14.12, 23.93) minutes	26.00 (95% CI, 15.48, 36.52) minutes	7.61 (95% CI, 0.51, 15.74) minutes (marginally improved)	9.91% (95% CI, 8.09%, 11.73%)	ISQ: 12.35 points (95% CI, 8.28–16.43 points) PSQI: 2.31 points (95% CI, 0.38–4.24 points)	20 studies (1162 participants [64% female; mean age, 56 y])
van Straten et al,[12] 2018	CBT-I or at least 1 component of it (individual, group or self-help)	Primary and comorbid insomnia	ES 0.57 (95% CI, 0.50, 0.65)	ES 0.63 (95% CI, 0.53, 0.73)	ES 0.16 (95% CI, 0.08, 0.24)	ES 0.71 (95% CI, 0.61, 0.82)	ISI: ES 0.98 (95% CI, 0.82–1.15) PSQI: ES 0.65 (95% CI, 0.51–0.79)	87 studies, including 6303 patients ES: Hedges' g
Wu et al,[15] 2015	CBT-I (in variations)	for comorbid insomnia (with psychiatric and medical conditions)	ES 0.80 (95% CI, 0.60, 1.00)	ES 0.68 (95% CI, 0.60, 0.98)	ES 0.19 (95% CI, 0.06, 0.31)	ES 0.91 (95% CI, 0.74, 1.08)	ES 0.84 (95% CI, 0.69–1.00)	37 trials reported with total 2189 participants; ES: Hedges' g

(continued on next page)

Table 1
(continued)

Treatment Format	Specific Program Features	Improvement in Sleep-onset Sleep-onset Latency, Post-treatment	Improvement in Wake Time After Sleep Onset, Post-treatment	Improvement in Total Sleep Time, Post-treatment	Improvement in Sleep Efficiency, Post-treatment	Subjective Sleep Quality, Post-treatment	Notes
Zachariae et al,[10] 2016	Internet based CBT-I: eCBT-I	(a) A multicomponent cognitive behavioral intervention for insomnia (CBT-I), including a combination of 2 or more elements typically considered part of CBT-I (sleep restriction, stimulus-control, cognitive therapy, sleep hygiene education, relaxation), (b) delivered over the Internet	ES 0.41 (95% CI, 0.29, 0.53)	ES 0.45 (95% CI, 0.25, 0.66)	ES 0.29 (95% CI, 0.17, 0.42)	ES 0.58 (95% CI, 0.36, 0.81)	ISI: ES 1.09 (95% CI, 0.74–1.45) 11 studies of 1460 participants (ES) Hedges' g

Abbreviations: e-CBT, Internet-based CBT; ISI, Insomnia Severity Index; ISQ, Insomnia Symptom Questionnaire; WL, Waitlist controls; WMD, Weighted mean difference.

meta-analyses, however, synthetized the remission rate from CBT-I. Compared with control groups, the remission rate of those receiving CBT-I is significantly higher (36% vs 16.9%).[15] Moreover, those who received CBT-I treatment were on average 2.89 times more likely to remit relative to those in inactive control groups.[16]

Although the benefits of CBT-I are well-established, few studies reported daytime function as an outcome measure despite its clinical significance and salience for the patient.[19] A recent meta-analysis[20] examined the effect of CBT-I or behavioral therapy (BT) for insomnia on depressive symptoms and daytime fatigue. Only individual, face-to-face CBT-I had a small to moderate effect on depressive symptoms (Cohen's d = 0.34; 95% CI, 0.06–0.63) but no significant effect on fatigue. Heterogeneities arising from treatment populations and symptom assessment, however, may have accounted for those findings. As suggested by the investigators, further studies are required to examine systematically treatment effects on daytime functioning of insomnia patients. The effect of CBT-I on daytime functioning is potentially confounded by some adverse effects from BT, especially with sleep restriction therapy (SRT).[21] Multiple side effects were reported by participants during the acute phase of SRT, with the 4 most common fatigue/exhaustion (100%), extreme sleepiness (94%), reduced motivation/energy (89%), and headache/migraine (72%). These adverse effects were positively associated with greater improvement on PSQI.[22] Nevertheless, the safety and efficacy of CBT-I warrant further research.[23]

Comparative Efficacy of Cognitive Behavioral Therapy for Insomnia and Sedative Hypnotics

The evidence on the comparative efficacy between CBT-I and sedative hypnotics is less well established. To the authors' knowledge, only 2 reviews have synthesized this body of evidence. In a meta-analysis of 21 studies,[24] the ESs of behavioral strategies (ie, stimulus control therapy and/or SRT) were evaluated against the short-term efficacy of BZDs and Z-drugs. Overall, moderate to large effects were observed across sleep measures for both types of therapies. Behavioral approaches were at least as effective as medications for improving SOL (ES SD 1.05 [0.76] vs 0.45 [0.28]), WASO (ES SD 1.03 [0.19] vs 0.89 [0.29]), and subjective sleep quality ratings (ES SD 1.44 [1.20] vs 1.20 [1.30]). On the other hand, medication was superior to BT in reducing the number of awakenings (ES 0.83 [1.30] vs 0.97 [1.00]) and increasing TST (ES 0.46 [0.62] vs ES 0.84 [0.76]). Due to the limited number of studies

directly comparing CBT-I with medications (n = 5), a more recent systematic review did not pool study findings but made comparisons between the 2 treatments using the grading of recommendations assessment, development and evaluation (GRADE) classification system.[25] Compared with medications, CBT-I demonstrated superior long-term (6–12 months) outcomes (low–moderate evidence) whereas medications produced better short-term (4–8 weeks) outcomes.[26] The extent to which these findings are applicable to emerging, self-help CBT-I formats or unique patient subpopulations is, however, unknown.

Cognitive Behavioral Therapy for Insomnia in Combination with Sedative Hypnotics

The theoretic premise for combining treatments is to capitalize on both the rapid symptomatic relief of sedative hypnotics and the sustained therapeutic benefits conferred by CBT-I (**Table 2**). Clinically, adding medication to CBT can potentially address adherence issues during the early course of CBT where tangible improvements are delayed by up to 4 weeks.[27] Combination therapies could also afford new opportunities for tailoring regimens that address interindividual differences in treatment response. Only a few clinical studies, however, have empirically investigated combined CBTI and sedative hypnotics.

Several studies show that the therapeutic benefits from the concomitant use of CBT-I and sedative hypnotics were not as sustainable as CBT-I alone. The therapeutic benefits from combined treatment declined in a similar pattern to the medication-only arm.[28–31] Such results may be explained by patients misattributing their sleep improvements to the sedative hypnotic exclusively and, therefore, may be at greater risk for relapse (ie, loss of therapeutic benefits) when medication is discontinued. The ease of use of sedative hypnotics may preclude an adequate opportunity for some patients to fully acquire the CBT-I skillset that would produce long-term therapeutic benefits. In 2 studies, however, the decline in therapeutic gains from combined treatment seemed mitigated by additional CBT-I booster sessions after the initial 5-week[32] and 6-month protocols,[23] respectively. Another approach for combining CBT-I and sedative hypnotics is through treatment sequencing. The optimal order for introducing medications and CBT-I components has been the subject of a recent clinical trial.[33] Preliminary findings show that initially, BTs produced higher remission rates than zolpidem (33% vs 25%). For the nonresponders of the respective groups, switching to a different treatment modality produced larger remission rates (eg, BT to zzolpidem).[34]

Table 2
The advantages and disadvantages of cognitive behavioral therapy for insomnia and pharmacotherapy

	Cognitive Behavioral Therapy for Insomnia	Pharmacotherapy
Advantages	• Teaches patients new skills to manage their sleep long term • Sustained therapeutic benefits • Patients feel more in control of their sleep • Few adverse effects relative to sedative hypnotics	• Rapid symptomatic relief • Requires little effort from patients
Disadvantages	• Requires motivation and high level of patient effort • Adherence may be challenging for some patients • Delayed therapeutic benefits • Experience of fatigue when initiating behavioral treatment, such as SRT	• Little evidence of long-term benefits and no evidence of sustained benefits after drug discontinuation • Potential for dependence, tolerance, and rebound insomnia • Side effects profile: sedation, memory loss

TREATMENT ACCEPTABILITY AND PREFERENCES

Whether a patient is treated with medication or CBT often is not determined by the evidence on treatment efficacy but is more dependent on who the patient sees in practice, that is, physician, psychologist, or other health care provider. The use and nonuse of pharmacotherapy in the management of insomnia has historically been an important issue both within sleep medicine and broader public health and safety. Alignment of treatment recommendations with patient preferences has been a longstanding pillar of patient-centered care because it influences patients' propensity and ability to initiate and adhere to treatment.[35,36] The latter is particularly important in the context of CBT-I because its effectiveness as a treatment is highly dependent on patient adherence to the prescribed protocol. Yet, how patient preferences situate between CBT-I and sleep medications remains inconclusive, and clinical and sociodemographic covariates do not reliably predict preference for the respective treatment options. Part of the misalignment stems from clinical research and practice, which operationalizes preference as a dichotomous outcome (ie, CBT-I vs sedative hypnotic) when these choices are not necessarily mutually exclusive.[37,38] Drawing from the qualitative literature, patients often attribute the cause of their insomnia as multifactorial (ie, biological, lifestyle, and age-related factors) and

welcome the idea of a triangulated approach of combining treatments.[38–40] Given the relationship between patients' illness beliefs and treatment needs, these findings make a compelling case for further developing protocols, which combine CBT-I with sedative hypnotics as part of the broader insomnia treatment plan.

Conceptually, treatment preference is the outcome of a decision-making process where patients deliberate between the merits and limitations of the respective options.[41] Because patients often formulate their understanding of treatments around psychosocial domains (relationship status, family commitments, and so forth) and illness beliefs, the upstream decision-making process that precedes preference can provide important insight for what patients prioritize along with the compromises they are willing to make. Reconceptualizing patient preferences on a continuum, therefore, can provide a novel gateway for improving the way clinicians engage with patients to understand their treatment needs. One novel application is through a shared decision framework that helps patients understand the merits and limitations of prospective treatments and make informed decisions about their insomnia care.

TYPICAL TRAJECTORY OF INSOMNIA HELP SEEKING

The previous sections highlight the current evidence for pharmacotherapy, CBT-I, and combined approaches, but beyond the evidence are several issues at the practice interface, which hinder research translation. Among these, delayed medical help seeking in favor of self-treatment is a well-established phenomenon.[42] Common reasons for not seeking medical care include the belief that insomnia is a self-limiting condition that will resolve, lack of awareness about treatment availability, and perceiving treatments as unattractive/ineffective.[43] Importantly, many of the self-help strategies implemented (eg, alcohol and herbal remedies) are not evidence based and may further contribute to perpetuating insomnia. Medical help-seeking is often triggered by the presence of daytime functional deficits.[44] Importantly, patients intuitively consult their primary care doctor for medical advice who are less attuned to psychotherapies than a psychologist. Furthermore, up to 90% of consultations end with a prescribed sedative hypnotic,[45] which may partly be driven by the time constraints of practice but also the assumption that patients only want a quick fix.[37,45] Together, optimizing insomnia treatments at the practice interface is met with several systemic challenges, such as tentative referral pathways in primary care, limited and uneven distribution of service providers,[46] and high up-front costs of CBT-I. The application of stepped care to the insomnia care pathway has been an important movement for the field to start resolving some of the aforementioned challenges. Stepped care organizes CBT-I resources into different levels of care and allocates patients to different levels of care based on insomnia severity to cost-effectively increase patient reach while conserving limited CBT-I specialist resources. Several issues remain unresolved, however, at the practice interface and are discussed later.[47]

TREATMENT AVAILABILITY AND GAPS IN CURRENT PRACTICE

Because the family physician is usually the first point of contact the patient engages with in the health care system, treatment is often limited to a prescribed medication. Despite this common practice, the family physician is well placed to initiate and/or triage the patient to some forms of abbreviated CBT-I programs, which tend to capitalize on the potentially underutilized front-line personnel and care venues. Such low-intensity interventions include brief behavioral treatment of insomnia,[48] dCBT-I programs,[49] or group CBT-I programs that run within the practice by a community nurse.[50] There seems, however, limited uptake of these treatment models into routine practice, where insomnia management continues to be restricted to the use of prescribed a sleeping pill and/or sleep hygiene in primary care.[51,52]

One reason for this research-practice gap is that these abbreviated CBT-I programs mostly have been evaluated in research/academic settings with limited transferability to routine practice that have operational constraints. Fortunately, several studies have started to address CBT-I implementation from a translational perspective, such as dCBT-I implanted in a primary care mental health setting.[53] Similarly, a pragmatic clinical trial is currently under way and being conducted by Morin and colleagues (clinicaltrials.gov: NCT03633305; https://clinicaltrials.gov/ct2/show/NCT03633305) to mimic a stepped care triage system in primary care. The trial design forgoes the randomization process to allow patients to select their preferred treatment after being informed about the risks (eg, adverse effects) and benefits of prospective treatment options through a shared decision-making framework. Patients initially receive self-help, dCBT-I or treatment as usual (typically no treatment or medication), or a combination of both. Those who do not remit from initial treatment are introduced to face-to-face CBT-I delivered by a psychologist or to a different medication than the one used during the initial-stage therapy. The integration of treatment preferences into the study design is based on the premise of patient engagement and understanding of treatment being critical for perceived self-efficacy and subsequent treatment adherence and optimize outcomes.

The scalability and potential reach of dCBT-I make it an appealing and cost-effective alternative to traditional CBT-I. One meta-analysis showed, however, that sleep improvements derived from this mode of treatment delivery are not well maintained at follow-up.[10] Furthermore, high attrition and poor adherence continue to be a burgeoning issue to be addressed, with the average dropout rate for dCBT-I programs reported at 24.7% (range 0.0%–41.3%).[10] Unfortunately, there were few studies discussing factors associated with dropout/completion of dCBT-I programs and it is further confounded by using noncompletion of post-assessment surveys as a proxy for noncompletion of the intervention. Nonetheless, with the continued expansion and iterations of CBT-I, broader applications of this intervention are expected to address common comorbidities and refractory cases presenting to clinical practice.

THE WHO AND HOW OF DISSEMINATING COGNITIVE BEHAVIORAL THERAPY FOR INSOMNIA

Given the shortage of sleep specialists in medical care, especially behavioral sleep medicine specialists, there is a need to train front-line personnel at different levels of practice (eg, social workers, nurses, pharmacists, psychologist, and psychiatrists) to allow CBT-I to be widely disseminated. There are inherent challenges, however, to training CBT-I providers from diverse disciplinary backgrounds. In a recent article, Manber and colleagues[54] discuss practical issues for developing materials and training nonspecialists in CBT-I within the Veterans Health Administration. Discussions centered on the competing demands that need to be considered at the practice interface, for example, program structure that ensures fidelity of content delivery while affording enough flexibility for the program to be adapted to different clinical experiences and practice constraints (eg, limited time, disruptions workload/workflow, and reimbursement structures). Key recommendations from the pilot training protocol included the need to target common presenting comorbidities in the practice environment (eg, posttraumatic stress disorder [PTSD], obstructive sleep apnea, and alcohol use in the Veterans Health Administration), adopting a semistructured treatment format that is useful for a potentially heterogenous patient population (eg, different patient preparedness for SRT), and strategic use of patient handouts to limit cognitive load. Case conceptualization was also considered a pragmatic means for teaching nonspecialists to identify and address causative factors of poor sleep. Although competency-based training and evaluation provided systematic way to impart knowledge to nonspecialists over a short period of 1.5 days, the need for more time to assimilate didactic and experiential components of training raises an important point of consideration in future program development.

THE CASE OF THE TREATMENT-RESISTANT PATIENT

Despite the extent of the evidence supporting the efficacy of CBT-I, used alone or in combination with pharmacotherapy, and the fact that a large majority of patients benefit from therapy, approximately 20% to 25% of patients do not respond to treatment. So, what can be done to address the needs of this insomnia patient subpopulation? Researchers have already proposed different approaches to tackle this problem. From a sleep physiology perspective, intensive sleep retraining (ISR) might provide a promising alternative for treatment resistant cases of insomnia. An ISR protocol rapidly builds sleep pressure where individuals are woken up 2 minutes to 3 minutes after entering stage 1 sleep at 30-minute intervals across a 24-hour period. The repeated rapid

sleep-wake cycles occurring over 24 hours essentially amount to several weeks of compliant stimulus control therapy.[45] From a psychological and emotional regulation perspective, incorporating acceptance and commitment therapy/ mindfulness approaches into CBT-I could play an important role in helping the individual accept unpleasant thoughts, feelings, and physical sensations, which often are perpetuated when an individual actively tries to eliminate these sensations. Likewise, acceptance and commitment therapy might be helpful at the end of therapy to assist patients in developing some tolerance for residual sleep disturbances, which are common even after successful CBT. Instilling behavioral and emotional flexibility may be especially important for nonresponders to treatment.[55] Population-based interventions to prevent insomnia also have gained attraction, targeting high-risk patient groups who are vulnerable to developing insomnia. This has given rise to low-intensity sleep health interventions using improved sleep as a way to mitigate the development of anxiety and depression among young adults.[56]

IMPACT OF EVIDENCE-BASED THERAPIES AND TREATMENT GUIDELINES ON CLINICAL PRACTICE

There are literally several hundred randomized clinical trials documenting the benefits of CBT-I with different groups of patients (younger and older adults), with or without comorbidities (eg, depression and pain), and using different treatment delivery methods (face-to-face, group, self-help, and digital). Based on this extensive outcome evidence, several professional sleep and medical associations have published clinical practice guidelines on the management of insomnia, including guidelines by the American College of Physicians,[2] the European Sleep Research Society,[1] and the AASM.[7] A common recommendation in all these guidelines is that CBT should be the first-line therapy for chronic insomnia, and only when such therapy is not available or not effective should medications be considered and only after addressing the potential harms and benefits of such therapy directly with the patient. Whether such a unified position statement coming from both the medical profession and professional sleep organizations will change clinical practices has yet to be documented. Likewise, despite the strong levels of evidence and professional endorsement for CBT-I, there is no guarantee that it will help overcome the common barriers (ie, cost and availability) to implementing

CBT-I in day-to-day clinical practices. Additional efforts are needed to disseminate further both the empirical evidence and practice guidelines to potential users.

SUMMARY

The field of insomnia treatment research has evolved tremendously over the past several decades. Pharmacologic research has moved from studying agents with a generalized central nervous system depressant effect, and all the adverse events such agents may produce, to studying molecules targeting more specific brain receptors and various release formulations to match insomnia subtypes (early, middle, and late insomnia). Likewise, the psychological literature has moved away from a narrow therapeutic approach comparing single interventions (eg, relaxation, stimulus control, and sleep restriction) to a more global, multifaceted approach incorporating cognitive, behavioral, and educational components, each targeting specific insomnia perpetuating factors. There also has been an important paradigm shift in which insomnia was previously conceptualized as a symptom of other psychiatric disorders to a conceptual framework in which insomnia can be diagnosed as a disorder of its own. Despite these advances in diagnosis and therapy, there is clearly room for further improvements because not all patients remit even with the best evidence-based therapies. Key areas for future research include

- Examination of optimal treatment algorithms, with or without medications, to determine what should be the first treatment and how to proceed with second-stage therapy for nonresponders
- Evaluation of personalized therapies based on patient preferences and insomnia phenotypes
- Validation of e-treatment delivery models— Web-based, mobile applications, and tele-health/medicine—to identify who is a good candidate for these self-guided, low-intensity models of care
- Investigation of new therapies for treatment-resistant cases (eg, ISR) and for patients with major psychiatric disorders

In addition to these research endeavors, finding more efficient methods is needed, to disseminate the best evidence-based therapies to potential users, that is, patients and clinicians, and increase lobbying efforts with government officials to improving access to psychological treatment of insomnia, similar to the UK National Health Service program, Adult Improving Access to Psychological Therapies programme (for anxiety and depression).

ACKNOWLEDGMENTS

Preparation of this article was supported in part by a grant from the Canadian Institutes of Health Research (#353509). Charles Morin has served as a consultant for Merck, Cereve, Abbott, and Phillips. The other authors did not declare any conflict.

REFERENCES

1. Riemann D, Baglioni C, Bassetti C, et al. European guideline for the diagnosis and treatment of insomnia. J Sleep Res 2017;26(6):675–700.
2. Qaseem A, Kansagara D, Forciea M, et al, Clinical Guidelines Committee of the American College of Physicians. Management of chronic insomnia disorder in adults: a clinical practice guideline from the american college of physicians. Ann Intern Med 2016;165(2):125–33.
3. Neubauer DN. New and emerging pharmacotherapeutic approaches for insomnia. Int Rev Psychiatry 2014;26(2):214–24.
4. Kuriyama A, Honda M, Hayashino Y. Ramelteon for the treatment of insomnia in adults: a systematic review and meta-analysis. Sleep Med 2014;15(4):385–92.
5. Winkler A, Auer C, Doering BK, et al. Drug treatment of primary insomnia: a meta-analysis of polysomnographic randomized controlled trials. CNS Drugs 2014;28(9):799–816.
6. Kuriyama A, Tabata H. Suvorexant for the treatment of primary insomnia: a systematic review and meta-analysis. Sleep Med Rev 2017;35:1–7.
7. Sateia MJ, Buysse DJ, Krystal AD, et al. Clinical practice guideline for the pharmacologic treatment of chronic insomnia in adults: an American Academy of Sleep Medicine clinical practice guideline. J Clin Sleep Med 2017;13(2):307–49.
8. Everitt H, Baldwin DS, Stuart B, et al. Antidepressants for insomnia in adults. Cochrane Database Syst Rev 2018;(5):CD010753.
9. Leach MJ, Page AT. Herbal medicine for insomnia: a systematic review and meta-analysis. Sleep Med Rev 2015;24:1–12.
10. Zachariae R, Lyby MS, Ritterband LM, et al. Efficacy of internet-delivered cognitive-behavioral therapy for insomnia - a systematic review and meta-analysis of randomized controlled trials. Sleep Med Rev 2016;30:1–10.
11. Koffel EA, Koffel JB, Gehrman PR. A meta-analysis of group cognitive behavioral therapy for insomnia. Sleep Med Rev 2015;19:6–16.

12. van Straten A, van der Zweerde T, Kleiboer A, et al. Cognitive and behavioral therapies in the treatment of insomnia: a meta-analysis. Sleep Med Rev 2018; 38:3–16.

13. Ho FYY, Chan CS, Tang KNS. Cognitive-behavioral therapy for sleep disturbances in treating posttraumatic stress disorder symptoms: a meta-analysis of randomized controlled trials. Clin Psychol Rev 2016;43:90–102.

14. Johnson JA, Rash JA, Campbell TS, et al. A systematic review and meta-analysis of randomized controlled trials of cognitive behavior therapy for insomnia (CBT-I) in cancer survivors. Sleep Med Rev 2016;27:20–8.

15. Wu JQ, Appleman ER, Salazar RD, et al. Cognitive behavioral therapy for insomnia comorbid with psychiatric and medical conditions: a Meta-analysis. JAMA Intern Med 2015;175(9):1461–72.

16. Brasure M, Fuchs E, MacDonald R, et al. Psychological and behavioral interventions for managing insomnia disorder: an evidence report for a clinical practice guideline by the American College of Physicians. Ann Intern Med 2016;165(2): 113–24.

17. Geiger-Brown JM, Rogers VE, Liu W, et al. Cognitive behavioral therapy in persons with comorbid insomnia: a meta-analysis. Sleep Med Rev 2015; 23:54–67.

18. Trauer JM, Qian MY, Doyle JS, et al. Cognitive behavioral therapy for chronic insomnia: a systematic review and meta-analysis. Ann Intern Med 2015;163(3):191–204.

19. Kyle SD, Morgan K, Espie CA. Insomnia and health-related quality of life. Sleep Med Rev 2010;14(1): 69–82.

20. Ballesio A, Aquino M, Feige B, et al. The effectiveness of behavioural and cognitive behavioural therapies for insomnia on depressive and fatigue symptoms: a systematic review and network meta-analysis. Sleep Med Rev 2018;37:114–29.

21. Kyle SD, Miller CB, Rogers Z, et al. Sleep restriction therapy for insomnia is associated with reduced objective total sleep time, increased daytime somnolence, and objectively impaired vigilance: implications for the clinical management of insomnia disorder. Sleep 2014;37(2):229–37.

22. Kyle SD, Morgan K, Spiegelhalder K, et al. No pain, no gain: an exploratory within-subjects mixed-methods evaluation of the patient experience of sleep restriction therapy (SRT) for insomnia. Sleep Med 2011;12(8):735–47.

23. Morin CM, Vallières A, Guay B, et al. Cognitive behavioral therapy, singly and combined with medication, for persistent insomnia: a randomized controlled trial. JAMA 2009;301(19):2005–15.

24. Smith MT, Perlis ML, Park A, et al. Comparative meta-analysis of pharmacotherapy and behavior therapy for persistent insomnia. Am J Psychiatry 2002;159(1):5–11.

25. GRADE Working Group. Grading quality of evidence and strength of recommendations. BMJ 2004; 328(7454):1490.

26. Mitchell M, Gehrman P, Perlis M, et al. Comparative effectiveness of cognitive behavioral therapy for insomnia: a systematic review. BMC Fam Pract 2012;13:40.

27. Morin CM, Espie C. Insomnia: a clinical guide to assessment and treatment. New York: Springer US; 2004.

28. Hauri PJ. Can we mix behavioral therapy with hypnotics when treating insomniacs? Sleep 1997; 20(12):1111–8.

29. Jacobs GD, Pace-Schott EF, Stickgold R, et al. Cognitive behavior therapy and pharmacotherapy for insomnia: a randomized controlled trial and direct comparison. Arch Intern Med 2004;164(17): 1888–96.

30. Wu R, Bao J, Zhang C, et al. Comparison of sleep condition and sleep-related psychological activity after cognitive-behavior and pharmacological therapy for chronic insomnia. Psychother Psychosom 2006;75(4):220–8.

31. Morin CM, Colecchi C, Stone J, et al. Behavioral and pharmacological therapies for late-life insomnia: a randomized controlled trial. JAMA 1999;281(11): 991–9.

32. Vallières A, Morin CM, Guay B. Sequential combinations of drug and cognitive behavioral therapy for chronic insomnia: an exploratory study. Behav Res Ther 2005;43(12):1611–30.

33. Morin CM, Edinger JD, Krystal AD, et al. Sequential psychological and pharmacological therapies for comorbid and primary insomnia: study protocol for a randomized controlled trial. Trials 2016;17(118):1–12.

34. Morin CM, Edinger JD, Krystal AD, et al. Sequential therapies for comorbid and primary insomnia: a randomized controlled trial. Sleep 2017;40(suppl_1): A127.

35. Morin CM, Gaulier B, Barry T, et al. Patients' acceptance of psychological and pharmacological therapies for insomnia. Sleep 1992;15(4):302–5.

36. Vincent N, Lewycky S, Finnegan H. Barriers to engagement in sleep restriction and stimulus control in chronic insomnia. J Consult Clin Psychol 2008; 76(5):820–8.

37. Dyas JV, Apekey TA, Tilling M, et al. Patients' and clinicians' experiences of consultations in primary care for sleep problems and insomnia: a focus group study. Br J Gen Pract 2010;60(574):e180–200.

38. Bluestein D, Healey AC, Rutledge CM. Acceptability of behavioral treatments for insomnia. J Am Board Fam Med 2011;24(3):272–80.

39. Cheung JMY, Bartlett DJ, Armour CL, et al. To drug or not to drug: a qualitative study of patients'

decision-making processes for managing insomnia. Behav Sleep Med 2018;16(1):1–26.

40. Cheung JMY, Bartlett DJ, Armour CL, et al. Insomnia patients' help-seeking experiences. Behav Sleep Med 2014;12(2):106–22.

41. Sidani S, Epstein DR, Bootzin RR, et al. Assessment of preferences for treatment: validation of a measure. Res Nurs Health 2009;32(4):419–31.

42. Morin CM, LeBlanc M, Daley M, et al. Epidemiology of insomnia: prevalence, self-help treatments, consultations, and determinants of help-seeking behaviors. Sleep Med 2006;7(2):123–30.

43. Stinson K, Tang NKY, Harvey AG. Barriers to treatment seeking in primary insomnia in the United Kingdom: a cross-sectional perspective. Sleep 2006;29(12):1643–6.

44. Aikens JE, Rouse ME. Help-seeking for insomnia among adult patients in primary care. J Am Board Fam Pract 2005;18(4):257–61.

45. Miller CB, Valenti L, Harrison CM, et al. Time trends in the family physician management of insomnia: the Australian experience (2000–2015). J Clin Sleep Med 2017;13(6):785–90.

46. Thomas A, Grandner M, Nowakowski S, et al. Where are the behavioral sleep medicine providers and where are they needed? a geographic assessment. Behav Sleep Med 2016;14(6):687–98.

47. Espie CA. "Stepped Care": a health technology solution for delivering cognitive behavioral therapy as a first line insomnia treatment. Sleep 2009;32(12):1549–58.

48. Buysse DJ, Germain A, Moul DE, et al. Efficacy of brief behavioral treatment for chronic insomnia in older adults. Arch Intern Med 2011;171(10):887–95.

49. Thorndike FP, Saylor DK, Bailey ET, et al. Development and perceived utility and impact of an internet intervention for insomnia. E J Appl Psychol 2008;4(2):32–42.

50. Espie CA, MacMahon KM, Kelly H-L, et al. Randomized clinical effectiveness trial of nurse-administered small-group cognitive behavior therapy for persistent insomnia in general practice. Sleep 2007;30(5):574–84.

51. van Rijswijk E, Borghuis M, van de Lisdonk E, et al. Treatment of mental health problems in general practice: a survey of psychotropics prescribed and other treatments provided. Int J Clin Pharmacol Ther 2007;45(1):23–9.

52. Everitt H, McDermott L, Leydon G, et al. GPs' management strategies for patients with insomnia: a survey and qualitative interview study. Br J Gen Pract 2014;64(619):e112–9.

53. Feuerstein S, Hodges S, Keenaghan B, et al. Computerized cognitive behavioral therapy for insomnia in a community health setting. J Clin Sleep Med 2017;13(2):267–74.

54. Manber R, Carney C, Edinger J, et al. Dissemination of CBTI to the non-sleep specialist: protocol development and training issues. J Clin Sleep Med 2012;8(2):209–18.

55. Dalrymple KL, Fiorentino L, Politi MC, et al. Incorporating principles from acceptance and commitment therapy into cognitive-behavioral therapy for insomnia: a case example. J Contemp Psychother 2010;40(4):209–17.

56. Werner-Seidler A, O'Dea B, Shand F, et al. A smartphone app for adolescents with sleep disturbance: development of the sleep ninja. JMIR Ment Health 2017;4(3):e28.

Cognitive Behavioral Therapy for Insomnia and Acute Insomnia
Considerations and Controversies

Jason G. Ellis, PhD

KEYWORDS

• Acute insomnia • Insomnia disorder • One-Shot • CBT-I

KEY POINTS

- The term "acute insomnia" has been part of the language of sleep medicine since the late 1970s.
- Despite that, a comprehensive research agenda on the topic has only recently been advanced.
- This has, at least until now, prevented a clinical viewpoint on the assessment and management of acute insomnia.
- Although there is a CBT-I-focused intervention designed to circumvent the transition from acute insomnia to insomnia disorder, the results from the trials undertaken have been variable and limited by small sample sizes.
- The findings from the review suggest there is still much work to be done with regard to the assessment, diagnosis, and management of acute insomnia.

INTRODUCTION
What is Acute Insomnia?

Before discussing the treatment of acute insomnia, within a cognitive behavioral therapy for insomnia (CBT-I) framework, it is appropriate to provide a working definition of the concept. When attempting to differentiate between what makes as case of any specific disease or disorder, or not, there are three perspectives to work from: (1) nosology, (2) theory, and (3) empirical work. In many instances, these three work in tandem, with new insights in each domain influencing the other two. However, that has been limited with respect to acute insomnia.

The nosologic perspective
The term "acute insomnia" was first listed in the International Classification of Diseases (ICD) in 1977.

This was followed by the American Sleep Disorders Association in 1979 and Diagnostic and Statistical Manual of Mental Disorders (DSM) in 1987. As time progressed and as the definition of insomnia disorder changed, so did the definition of acute insomnia (otherwise known as short-term insomnia, transient insomnia, adjustment insomnia, or stress-related insomnia). Currently, the ICD-10 identifies acute insomnia under the framework of meeting all the criteria for nonorganic insomnia, except duration (ie, not being present for at least 1 month).[1] Both the International Classification of Sleep Disorders–3rd Edition[2] and DSM-5[3] follow the same logic as the ICD-10, in that, acute insomnia is defined based on not meeting the duration criterion for insomnia disorder (however, in these instances 3 months). In fact, the DSM-5 explicitly states that if all other criteria are met, except duration, it is to be defined as acute, or

Funding: This study was in part funded by the Economic and Social Research Council (RES-061-25-0120-A). The funders had no role in any aspect of the study or production of the article.
Northumbria Sleep Research Laboratory, Faculty of Health and Life Sciences, Northumbria University, 134/408 Northumberland Building, Newcastle upon Tyne NE1 8ST, UK
E-mail address: Jason.ellis@northumbria.ac.uk

Sleep Med Clin 14 (2019) 267–274
https://doi.org/10.1016/j.jsmc.2019.01.007
1556-407X/19/Crown Copyright © 2019 Published by Elsevier Inc. All rights reserved.

short-term, insomnia with a specific classification of "another specified insomnia disorder."[3] Therefore, within each framework, acute insomnia has largely been defined based on not meeting criteria for insomnia disorder. This leads to the first consideration regarding its assessment and management. When does acute insomnia become insomnia disorder and when should it be managed? Working from the current nosologies, acute insomnia is defined based on having insomnia disorder for less than 1 or 3 months. It is unclear, however, on what basis the current duration criteria for insomnia disorder originated. Previous iterations of the DSM, the ICD, and International Classification of Sleep Disorders have outlined differing duration criteria with some going as far as 6 months. Conversely, is insomnia experienced for 1 week, or 2 weeks, still acute insomnia? In essence, what changes should one expect to see that signify the beginning and end of acute insomnia? Where this is not outlined explicitly in any nosology, and there is a limited evidence base in this area, there is one suggestion embedded within many of the models of insomnia.

The theoretic perspective

Spielman's model of insomnia is, arguably, the first model of insomnia that outlines the trajectory of insomnia from its premorbid to chronic state.[4–6] Regarding acute insomnia, Spielman suggests that the precipitant (ie, a major life event), which may be biologic or social in nature, is the main driver of insomnia before its transition to insomnia disorder. Although the idea that acute insomnia has to be driven by a major life event has been questioned with respect to the accumulation of daily hassles and/or chronic stress[7,8] as triggers, the idea of the precipitant being the driver of acute insomnia has remained central to the models that followed Spielman (eg, Perlis and colleagues,[9]

Harvey,[10] Lundh and Broman,[11] Perlstrom and Wickramasekera,[12] Buysse and colleagues[13]). The only model that explicitly outlines the trajectory from normal sleep to acute insomnia is from Espie.[14] Like Spielman, Espie suggests that acute insomnia originates from a stressor and during the acute phase it is the impact of the stressor that determines the resultant sleep disturbance. Furthermore, Espie signifies the transition to insomnia disorder when the source of the stress changes to sleep as opposed to the stressor itself and manifests through increased attention to sleep and focused intention and increased effort to regain sleep. One of the challenges of the existing models is that although they may specify a specific change that signifies the transition from acute insomnia to insomnia disorder, such as Espie does, none provide a timeline for when this change might occur, nor how this could be measured.

This stress-diathesis perspective outlined in each of the insomnia models also leads to a second consideration. If acute insomnia manifests in response to a precipitant event, and perpetuating factors are not altogether evident during this phase, why would a CBT-I framework be an appropriate treatment strategy? The central tenet of CBT-I is to identify and manage sleep-related dysfunctional thoughts, feelings, and behaviors (ie, perpetuating factors), with the precipitant usually ignored within the framework of CBT-I. Therefore, if it were the case that perpetuating factors are minimal, if evident at all, during the acute phase then it would stand to reason that a stress-reduction-based treatment strategy would be a more meaningful and effective candidate. That said, a careful examination of Spielman's model demonstrates two stages where the insomnia threshold has been breached but is not at the point of insomnia disorder (**Fig. 1**), the latter stage of which suggests the introduction of perpetuating factors, albeit minimally.

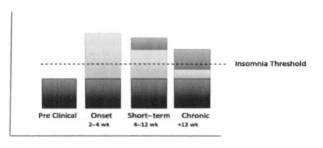

Fig. 1. Spielman's 3P model of insomnia, with proposed timeline.

The empirical perspective Without a consensus definition or a model that outlines a specific timeline within which to examine acute insomnia, its study has been limited.[15] Most research that has been undertaken has been in an attempt to understand the pathophysiology of insomnia disorder using a stressor as an analogue for acute insomnia. Various methods have been used, such as physiologic (eg, caffeine supplementation, rapid change in sleep timing), environmental (eg, noise, light, and temperature), and psychological (eg, social stress test, complex cognitive tasks) challenge.[16–21] In each case the stressor used has been shown to disrupt sleep continuity and sleep architecture.[22,23]

The validity of these studies as an analogue for acute insomnia, or even insomnia disorder, however, is questionable. Most of these studies do not use a research protocol lasting a week with at least 3 nights of stress-related disruption. As such these studies do not meet the minimum frequency or, by design, duration criteria set out in any of the nosologies. It could also be argued that they are unlikely to meet criteria for daytime disorder or dysfunction because in most cases research participants are required, by ethics boards and committees, to have a period of recovery the day following the night of sleep disruption. Another consideration is with regard to the aspect of informed consent procedures. In most cases the subject in the study would have been informed that they were likely to face a stressor either before bed or in the morning. This does not fit with the phenomenology of insomnia, at least in terms of insomnia disorder, with respect to its perceived unpredictable nature.[24–26]

Based on the existing nosologies, the theories advanced by Spielman, Espie, and others, and the existing evidence Ellis and colleagues,[7] created a working definition of acute insomnia in 2012. This definition (**Table 1** for the full criteria) suggests that acute insomnia should be defined as a self-reported disruption in sleep continuity for between 2 weeks and 3 months in duration.

What is Known About Acute Insomnia?

Based on this definition, acute insomnia has a point prevalence of between 7.9% (United Kingdom) and 9.5% (United States) and for just more than half of those reporting acute insomnia (51.2%) it is reported as a first episode. Furthermore, the annual incidence of acute insomnia is in the region of 31% to 36%.[27]

The sleep of individuals with first-onset acute insomnia differs from that of normal sleepers. Subjectively, it differs in terms of increased time awake during the night (at sleep onset and over the

Table 1	
Diagnostic criteria for acute insomnia	
Principle Complaint	1. A self-reported difficulty in initiating or maintaining sleep, or early morning awakening 2. The problem should exist despite adequate opportunity for sleep
Trigger	1. A significant life event or a chronic stressor 2. A series of daily stressors
Associated features	1. Distress at current situation 2. A significant reduction in quality of life
Timeline	3–14 d: subacute 2–4 wk: acute 1–3 mo: subchronic
Qualitative criteria	Self-defined as: mild, moderate, or severe
Quantitative criteria	1. Sleep latency 30 or more min 2. Wake after sleep onset of 30 or more min

Data from Ellis JG, Gehrman P, Espie CA, et al. Acute insomnia: current conceptualizations and future directions. Sleep Med Rev 2012;16(1):5–14.

course of the night), a higher number of nocturnal awakenings, and a lower sleep efficiency.[28,29] Objectively, those with acute insomnia differ from normal sleepers in terms of higher sleep fragmentation at night via actigraphy,[28,29] and higher amounts of stage 2 (N2) sleep and lower amounts of slow wave sleep (N3) via polysomnography.[29] Furthermore, those with first-onset acute insomnia tend to show, in addition to these differences in subjective and objective sleep, a slight circadian delay in addition to decrements in daytime energy expenditure, broadly resembling a 90-minure cycle, most pronounced during the morning.[30] Importantly, none of the objective differences observed in these studies (ie, higher N2, lower N3) are generally seen in those with insomnia disorder,[31,32] suggesting that acute insomnia may be quantitatively different from full insomnia disorder. At this juncture, however, it is uncertain whether these differences are specific to acute insomnia in general, or whether they only present during the first episode of any form of insomnia.

In terms of other differences between individuals with acute insomnia and those with insomnia disorder there is one cross-sectional study that compared groups on individual differences in coping styles.[33] The main finding from that study was that those with acute insomnia used self-punishment as a strategy to deal with unwanted intrusive thoughts, more so than those with insomnia disorder. That said, because the study used a duration criteria of 6 months to differentiate the groups, it is unknown how these data fit with the current definition of acute insomnia.

What is Known About the Transition from Acute Insomnia to Insomnia Disorder?

Subjective sleep continuity data during the first episode do not differ between those with acute insomnia who go on to develop insomnia disorder and those who naturally remit.[29] However, those who transition to insomnia disorder demonstrate two differences in their sleep architecture compared with normal sleepers and those who would naturally remit.[29] Those who would go on to develop insomnia disorder showed a shorter rapid eye movement onset latency (mean minutes, 66.32) compared with normal sleepers (mean minutes, 92.69) and those who would remit (mean minutes, 97.08) at baseline. Furthermore, lower amounts of N3 (6.51% of total sleep) compared with normal sleepers (16.99% of total sleep) were observed. Additionally, because the number of life events experienced over the previous year, stress levels over the previous month, nor current levels of anxiety and depression did not differ between those who would later remit and those who would develop insomnia disorder it is unlikely that these results could be explained as an epiphenomenon to the precipitating factors that triggered the insomnia. What these figures point to, especially the early onset of rapid eye movement, is a vulnerability for the onset of depression.[34,35] Again, however, it is unclear whether these are features of acute insomnia in general or specific to the first episode. Although this does not directly impact on the treatment choice for acute insomnia, what this does point to is the wider issue of the need to address acute insomnia because of the potential for the onset of depression.

There is one small study that compared individuals with acute insomnia against those with insomnia disorder in terms of sleep-related cognitions and behaviors, sleep-associated monitoring, perceived stress and worry, and objective (actigraphy) and subjective (sleep diary and Insomnia Severity Index) sleep.[36] Whereas differences between the groups were observed in terms of higher levels of stress being reported by those with acute insomnia, no differences between the groups in terms of sleep-incompatible cognitions and behaviors were evident. Albeit tentatively because of the sample size this finding suggests that perpetuating factors do have a role to play during acute insomnia (as defined based on meeting criteria for DSM-5 insomnia disorder between 2 weeks and 3 months in duration). A more recent study adds support to this idea, because sleep-related dysfunctional beliefs were a significant predictor of those who would transition to insomnia disorder within a 3-month window in a group of hospitalized individuals.[37] Based on these studies it seems that a CBT-I framework might be a treatment candidate for this population.

TREATING ACUTE INSOMNIA WITH COGNITIVE BEHAVIORAL THERAPY FOR INSOMNIA

Working from the premise that perpetuating factors are a feature of acute insomnia but are likely to be in their infancy, as suggested by Spielman, and brief therapies for insomnia, such as abbreviated CBT-I and brief behavioral therapy for insomnia, can effect change in individuals with insomnia disorder,[38–40] Ellis and colleagues[41] developed a "one-shot" CBT-I intervention specifically to prevent the transition from acute insomnia to insomnia disorder. To date, this is the only intervention that has been applied to this population. The intervention comprised a pamphlet and a single 60- to 70-minute face-to-face session. The rationale for a single session came from Edinger and coworkers,[42] who demonstrated that it is possible to front load CBT-I into a single session with good results. The rationale for the amount of contact time came from an examination of the previous brief therapies, which suggested approximately 60 minutes was sufficient to elicit change in individuals with insomnia disorder.[38,40,43]

The One-Shot Pamphlet

The pamphlet was framed as the 3Ds (Detect, Detach, and Distract) and was broadly aligned to two of the principle components contained within traditional CBT-I (ie, stimulus control and cognitive therapy). In addition, there was a brief description of acute insomnia (framed as stress-related sleep loss) and the suggestion that although it was unlikely that the bedroom environment caused the problem, if the bedroom were too hot or cold, too light or too noisy it could make the problem worse. The pamphlet contained four key points:

- How to record a sleep diary. The aim of the sleep diary was threefold: (1) as a method of recording patterns and changes in symptoms, (2) as a method to determine the sleep restriction prescription in the treatment session, and (3) something to be taken to a general practitioner if the individual did not wish to or could not attend a single session but would still like support for their insomnia. The instructions were focused on recording the main symptomology of insomnia: sleep latency, number of awakenings, wake after sleep onset, and the core elements needed to calculate sleep efficiency (time in bed and total sleep time). The diary was to be recorded every day for a minimum of 1 continuous week.

- Stimulus control instructions. Based on the original concepts of Bootzin and coworkers,[44] the aim was to recondition the relationship between the bedroom and sleep while simultaneously increasing the sleep drive. The instructions were to (1) only use the bedroom for sleep and sex, (2) leave the bedroom if unable to sleep, and (3) not to sleep in any other environment.

- Cognitive control instructions. The aim of this element was to reduce the potential for nocturnal rumination and worry by giving the individual a sense of control over their previous, and next, days activities. The instructions were to put the day to bed before the individual went to bed by creating a period of reflection (kept in the form of lists) a few hours before bedtime. This period involved reflecting on what the individual had achieved that day, what they had to do the following day, and what they had put into place to deal with the demands of the following day.

- Distraction techniques. As a form of articulatory suppression[45] the aim was to engage the individual with acute insomnia to address nocturnal intrusive thoughts using one of three techniques: (1) visual, (2) numeric, or (3) alphabetical. These techniques were designed to be meaningless but mentally consuming with the intention of overloading executive function in the brain.

The pamphlet was designed to be provided a week before the treatment session, alongside a sleep diary, so that the initial sleep prescription could be discussed during the single session.

The One-Shot Treatment Session

The single session outlines two further elements taken from traditional CBT-I; sleep-related psychoeducation and sleep restriction. The psychoeducation component involves a brief discussion, using pictorial versions of Spielman's 3P Model[4–6] and Borbély's[46] Two Process Model of sleep/wake regulation, on what insomnia is and why it occurs. The other aspect of this component involves a discussion on individual differences in sleep need throughout the lifespan. As with

traditional sleep restriction, total sleep time from the sleep diary is used to determine the prescribed sleep schedule over the following week (ie, total sleep time becomes time in bed). The individual, with help from the therapist, then agrees the morning anchor time and is then instructed to stick to the schedule for the next week. Next, the titration schedule for the following weeks, based on sleep efficiency, is discussed with the following rules: less than 85%, the individual goes to bed 15 minutes later for the next week; between 85% and 89%, the prescription stays the same for the next week; and more than 90%, the individual can go to bed 15 minutes earlier than previously for the next week. It is also reinforced that the individual should not reduce their time in bed to less than 5 hours, irrespective of what the sleep diary calculations suggest. Safeguarding in case of excessive daytime sleepiness is also discussed at this point. Finally, the time remaining is devoted to discussing potential barriers and solutions to the treatment.[47]

The Evidence for the One-Shot

There are currently three studies that have examined the impact of the One-Shot.[41,48,49] The first contained a feasibility study on the pamphlet alone in terms of reductions in cognitive and somatic tension (significant reductions on both domains were evident 1 week postdelivery) and randomized controlled trial of the full intervention.[41] The second study mirrored the first in that it was on a self-selecting community-based sample with the aim to determine whether the One Shot could be delivered in a group context and whether outcomes would differ based on individualized versus group treatment.[48] The third and final study looked at a particularly vulnerable population (prison inmates[49]) where rates of insomnia disorder are high (approximately 61%[50]) and the evidence suggests that the insomnia develops within that environment.[51]

The findings from each respective study have been promising in terms of remission rates and reductions in insomnia symptoms at 1-month posttreatment follow-ups (**Table 2**). In terms of adherence, using a rule of 15 minutes outside of prescribed sleep scheduled times during the first week of treatment being an indicator of nonadherence, 60% of those in the first study were adherent compared with 72.76% in the second study and 90% in the final study. As seen in **Table 2**, however, the effect sizes are variable between the first study and the second and third. There are several potential reasons for this including therapist factors, the inclusion of individuals with a range of

Table 2
Overview of study outcomes

Study	Sample Characteristics	Effect Sizes							One-Month Remission Rate (%)	Three-Month Remission Rate (%)
		ISI	SL	WASO	TST	SE	GAD-7	PHQ-9		
Ellis et al,[41] 2015	40 adults (55% female)	0.64	0.71	0.77	0.28	0.69	N/R	N/R	60	72
Boullin et al,[48] 2017	25 adults (76% female)	2.27	1.06	1.01	0.17	1.23	1.26	1.28	72.12	N/R
Randall et al,[49] 2018	30 male prisoners	2.35	1.49	0.93	0.87	0.91	0.83	0.77	73	N/R

Abbreviations: GAD-7, anxiety scores from the generalized anxiety disorder-7; ISI, insomnia severity index; N/R, not recorded; PHQ-9, depression from the patient health questionnaire-9 minus the sleep item; SE, sleep efficiency; SL, sleep latency; TST, total sleep time; WASO, wake after sleep onset.

chronic physical and/or psychological illnesses in the first study but not the other two, adherence rates, and/or the small sample sizes involved. These issues should be examined closely in further studies of the One Shot. There were no significant differences between group treatment versus individualized treatment, suggesting it can be delivered in groups (although those in groups were less adherent [53.85% vs 91.67%]). Furthermore, where the final two studies examined changes in anxiety and depression scores, significant reductions were evident in both cases.

THE FUTURE OF ACUTE INSOMNIA (ASSESSMENT AND MANAGEMENT)

Clearly there is still much work to be done in understanding the phenomenology of acute insomnia and its place within the pathophysiology of insomnia disorder. Although a definition now exists, this needs further empirical testing, especially with regard to the timing of the definition. Further testing of the One-Shot, in addition to other interventions aimed at acute insomnia, is also warranted. This is especially true when considering the slight circadian delay observed in individuals with acute insomnia, which is not yet featured in current treatment protocols. Another avenue is to address deployment, not only in terms of the One-Shot, but any intervention aimed at preventing insomnia disorder. Further research needs to be done with respect to what kinds of precipitants are more likely to trigger insomnia and what treatment-seeking behavior occurs at this time. Knowing more about the triggers could certainly inform delivery location (eg, job centers, bereavement counseling organizations) and early treatment-seeking behaviors may well provide

additional insights into delivery location (eg, primary care, pharmacy) that in turn can inform whom may be best placed to deliver the intervention.

Recently, Edinger and colleagues[52] showed poorer treatment outcomes, using pharmacotherapy or CBT-I, in those with insomnia disorder whose first episode of insomnia and depression occurred in childhood compared with those who developed both conditions, for the first time, in adulthood. That said, it could not be determined whether the poorer treatment response was caused by (1) the age of first onset, (2) the length of exposure to insomnia (first onset at 13.1 ± 5.27 year old for childhood onset vs 38.6 ± 12.2 year old for adult onset), or (3) the number of episodes of insomnia experienced (2.5 ± 3.05 vs 1.7 ± 2.38). This tentatively points to another area of future research with respect to the assessment and management of acute insomnia. Are there differences between first-onset acute insomnia and a recurrent episode of acute insomnia, which may require different treatment approaches? Finally, an examination of the relationship between sleep reactivity and acute insomnia may be fruitful, especially considering recent research that demonstrates that an episode of insomnia may impact on subsequent episodes.[53,54]

SUMMARY

The term acute insomnia has been part of the language of sleep medicine since the late 1970s. Despite that, a comprehensive research agenda on the topic has only recently been advanced. This has, at least until now, prevented a clinical viewpoint on the assessment and management of acute insomnia. Although there is a CBT-I-focused intervention designed to circumvent the transition from acute insomnia to insomnia disorder, the results from the trials undertaken have been variable and have been limited by small sample sizes. The findings from the review suggest there is still much work to be done with regard to the assessment, diagnosis, and management of acute insomnia.

REFERENCES

1. World Health Organization. The ICD-10 classification of mental and behavioural disorders: clinical descriptions and diagnostic guidelines, vol. 1. Geneva (Switzerland): World Health Organization; 1992.
2. American Academy of Sleep Medicine. International classification of sleep disorders–third edition (ICSD-3). Darien (IL): American Academy of Sleep Medicine; 2014.
3. American Psychiatric Association. Diagnostic and statistical manual of mental disorders (DSM-5). Washington, DC: American Psychiatric Pub; 2013.
4. Spielman AJ. Assessment of insomnia. Clin Psychol Rev 1986;6(1):11–25.
5. Spielman AJ, Caruso LS, Glovinsky PB. A behavioral perspective on insomnia treatment. Psychiatr Clin 1987;10(4):541–53.
6. Spielman AJ, Saskin P, Thorpy MJ. Treatment of chronic insomnia by restriction of time in bed. Sleep 1987;10(1):45–56.
7. Ellis JG, Gehrman P, Espie CA, et al. Acute insomnia: current conceptualizations and future directions. Sleep Med Rev 2012;16(1):5–14.
8. Morin CM, Rodrigue S, Ivers H. Role of stress, arousal, and coping skills in primary insomnia. Psychosom Med 2003;65(2):259–67.
9. Perlis ML, Giles DE, Mendelson WB, et al. Psychophysiological insomnia: the behavioural model and a neurocognitive perspective. J Sleep Res 1997; 6(3):179–88.
10. Harvey AG. A cognitive model of insomnia. Behav Res Ther 2002;40(8):869–93.
11. Lundh LG, Broman JE. Insomnia as an interaction between sleep-interfering and sleep-interpreting processes. J Psychosom Res 2000;49(5):299–310.
12. Perlstrom JR, Wickramasekera I. Insomnia, hypnotic ability, negative affectivity, and the high risk model of threat perception. J Nerv Ment Dis 1998;186(7):437–40.
13. Buysse DJ, Germain A, Hall M, et al. A neurobiological model of insomnia. Drug Discov Today Dis Models 2011;8(4):129–37.
14. Espie CA. Insomnia: conceptual issues in the development, persistence, and treatment of sleep disorder in adults. Annu Rev Psychol 2002;53(1):215–43.
15. Perlis ML, Gehrman P, Ellis JG. The natural history of insomnia: what we know, don't know, and need to know. Sleep Med Res 2011;2:79–88.
16. Zammit G, Schwartz H, Roth T, et al. The effects of ramelteon in a first-night model of transient insomnia. Sleep Med 2009;10(1):55–9.
17. Staner L, Eriksson M, Cornette F, et al. Sublingual zolpidem is more effective than oral zolpidem in initiating early onset of sleep in the post-nap model of transient insomnia: a polysomnographic study. Sleep Med 2009;10(6):616–20.
18. Paterson LM, Wilson SJ, Nutt DJ, et al. A translational, caffeine-induced model of onset insomnia in rats and healthy volunteers. Psychopharmacology 2007;191(4):943–50.
19. Bonnet MH, Arand DL. Caffeine use as a model of acute and chronic insomnia. Sleep 1992;15(6): 526–36.
20. Stone BM, Turner C, Mills SL, et al. Noise-induced sleep maintenance insomnia: hypnotic and residual effects of zaleplon. Br J Clin Pharmacol 2002;53(2): 196–202.
21. Hall M, Thayer JF, Germain A, et al. Psychological stress is associated with heightened physiological arousal during NREM sleep in primary insomnia. Behav Sleep Med 2007;5(3):178–93.
22. Riemann D, Spiegelhalder K, Feige B, et al. The hyperarousal model of insomnia: a review of the concept and its evidence. Sleep Med Rev 2010; 14(1):19–31.
23. Bonnet MH, Arand DL. Hyperarousal and insomnia: state of the science. Sleep Med Rev 2010;14(1): 9–15.
24. Buysse DJ, Cheng Y, Germain A, et al. Night-to-night sleep variability in older adults with and without chronic insomnia. Sleep Med 2010;11(1):56–64.
25. Vallières A, Ivers H, Bastien CH, et al. Variability and predictability in sleep patterns of chronic insomniacs. J Sleep Res 2005;14(4):447–53.
26. Perlis ML, Swinkels CM, Gehrman PR, et al. The incidence and temporal patterning of insomnia: a pilot study. J Sleep Res 2010;19(1-Part-I):31–5.
27. Ellis JG, Perlis ML, Neale LF, et al. The natural history of insomnia: focus on prevalence and incidence of acute insomnia. J Psychiatr Res 2012;46(10): 1278–85.
28. Holloway PM, Angelova M, Lombardo S, et al. Complexity analysis of sleep and alterations with insomnia based on non-invasive techniques. J R Soc Interface 2014;11(93):20131112.
29. Ellis JG, Perlis ML, Bastien CH, et al. The natural history of insomnia: acute insomnia and first-onset depression. Sleep 2014;37(1):97–106.
30. Fossion R, Rivera AL, Toledo-Roy JC, et al. Multiscale adaptive analysis of circadian rhythms and intradaily variability: application to actigraphy time series in acute insomnia subjects. PLoS One 2017; 12(7):e0181762.
31. Feige B, Al-Shajlawi A, Nissen C, et al. Does REM sleep contribute to subjective wake time in primary

insomnia? A comparison of polysomnographic and subjective sleep in 100 patients. J Sleep Res 2008; 17(2):180–90.

32. Baglioni C, Regen W, Teghen A, et al. Sleep changes in the disorder of insomnia: a meta-analysis of polysomnographic studies. Sleep Med Rev 2014;18(3):195–213.

33. Ellis J, Cropley M. An examination of thought control strategies employed by acute and chronic insomniacs. Sleep Med 2002;3(5):393–400.

34. Perlis ML, Giles DE, Buysse DJ, et al. Self-reported sleep disturbance as a prodromal symptom in recurrent depression. J Affect Disord 1997;42(2–3): 209–12.

35. Perlis ML, Giles DE, Buysse DJ, et al. Which depressive symptoms are related to which sleep electroencephalographic variables? Biol Psychiatry 1997; 42(10):904–13.

36. Man S, Freeston M, Ellis JG, et al. A pilot study investigating differences in sleep and life preoccupations in chronic and acute insomnia. Sleep Med Res 2013;4(2):43–50.

37. Griffiths MF, Peerson A. Risk factors for chronic insomnia following hospitalization. J Adv Nurs 2005;49:245–53.

38. Germain A, Moul DE, Franzen PL, et al. Effects of a brief behavioral treatment for late-life insomnia: preliminary findings. J Clin Sleep Med 2006;2(04): 407–8.

39. McCrae CS, Bramoweth AD, Williams J, et al. Impact of brief cognitive behavioral treatment for insomnia on health care utilization and costs. J Clin Sleep Med 2014;10(02):127–35.

40. Edinger JD, Sampson WS. A primary care "friendly" cognitive behavioral insomnia therapy. Sleep 2003; 26(2):177–82.

41. Ellis JG, Cushing T, Germain A. Treating acute insomnia: a randomized controlled trial of a "single-shot" of cognitive behavioral therapy for insomnia. Sleep 2015;38(6):971–8.

42. Edinger JD, Wohlgemuth WK, Radtke RA, et al. Dose-response effects of cognitive-behavioral insomnia therapy: a randomized clinical trial. Sleep 2007;30(2):203–12.

43. Lovato N, Lack L, Wright H, et al. Evaluation of a brief treatment program of cognitive behavior therapy for insomnia in older adults. Sleep 2014;37(1): 117–26.

44. Bootzin RR, Epstein D, Wood JM. Stimulus control instructions. In: Hauri P, editor. Case studies in insomnia. Boston: Springer; 1991. p. 19–28.

45. Levey AB, Aldaz JA, Watts FN, et al. Articulatory suppression and the treatment of insomnia. Behav Res Ther 1991;29(1):85–9.

46. Borbély AA. A two process model of sleep regulation. Hum Neurobiol 1982;1(3):195–204.

47. Miller CB, Espie CA, Epstein DR, et al. The evidence base of sleep restriction therapy for treating insomnia disorder. Sleep Med Rev 2014;18(5): 415–24.

48. Boullin P, Ellwood C, Ellis JG. Group vs. individual treatment for acute insomnia: a pilot study evaluating a "one-shot" treatment strategy. Brain Sci 2017;7(1):1.

49. Randall C, Nowakowski S, Ellis JG. Managing acute insomnia in prison: evaluation of a "one-shot" cognitive behavioral therapy for insomnia (CBT-I) intervention. Behav Sleep Med 2018;16(10):1–10.

50. Dewa LH, Kyle SD, Hassan L, et al. Prevalence, associated factors and management of insomnia in prison populations: an integrative review. Sleep Med Rev 2015;24:13–27.

51. Elger BS. Prevalence, types and possible causes of insomnia in a swiss remand prison. Eur J Epidemiol 2004;19:665–77.

52. Edinger JD, Manber R, Buysse DJ, et al. Are patients with childhood onset of insomnia and depression more difficult to treat than are those with adult onsets of these disorders? A report from the TRIAD study. J Clin Sleep Med 2017;13(2):205–13.

53. Jarrin DC, Chen IY, Ivers H, et al. The role of vulnerability in stress-related insomnia, social support and coping styles on incidence and persistence of insomnia. J Sleep Res 2014;23(6):681–8.

54. Kalmbach DA, Pillai V, Arnedt JT, et al. Sleep system sensitization: evidence for changing roles of etiological factors in insomnia. Sleep Med 2016;21:63–9.

Delivering Cognitive Behavioral Therapy for Insomnia in the Real World
Considerations and Controversies

Luis F. Buenaver, PhD[a],*, Donald Townsend, PhD[b],
Jason C. Ong, PhD[c]

KEYWORDS

- Insomnia • Cognitive behavioral therapy for insomnia • Stimulus control • Sleep restriction • CBT-I

KEY POINTS

- Cognitive behavioral therapy for insomnia (CBT-I) is recommended as the first-line treatment of insomnia but barriers remain in the implementation of CBT-I in the health care system.
- Delivery of CBT-I now includes scalable formats, such as Internet-based delivery, which improves accessibility but also raises questions regarding oversight and regulation of these treatment modalities.
- Although CBT-I has been shown to be effective, it remains unclear who is an appropriate candidate and what factors might serve as contraindications for CBT-I.
- The shift toward quality care among health care systems has produced a need for quality measures to evaluate the process and outcomes of delivering CBT-I.

INTRODUCTION

Insomnia is the most common sleep disorder in the general population and is characterized by difficulty with sleep onset, sleep maintenance, and/or nonrestorative sleep that results in daytime impairment. An accumulation of empirical evidence supporting the efficacy of cognitive behavioral therapy for insomnia (CBT-I) has resulted in the recommendation of CBT-I as a first-line treatment of adults with insomnia.[1–3] CBT-I is a multicomponent treatment featuring behavioral techniques designed to deepen and consolidate sleep, regularize sleep patterns, and elicit a physiologic relaxation response. Often, CBT-I also includes cognitive techniques designed to correct maladaptive thinking about sleep and sleep-related coping behaviors. Within the last decade, CBT-I has been used with various medical and psychiatric populations, such as cardiovascular disease,[4] osteoarthritis,[5] posttraumatic stress disorder,[6] depression,[7] and schizophrenia.[8] Despite broad acknowledgment of CBT-I's effectiveness, it remains massively underused relative to the large proportion of adults who suffer from chronic insomnia.

This article discusses the considerations and controversies involved in delivering CBT-I in the

Conflict of interest: None.
[a] Departments of Psychiatry and Behavioral Sciences, and Neurology, Johns Hopkins University School of Medicine, 5510 Nathan Shock Drive, Suite 100, Baltimore, MD 21224, USA; [b] Arizona School of Professional Psychology at Argosy University, 3322 West Dunlap Avenue, Phoenix, AZ 85021, USA; [c] Department of Neurology, Northwestern University Feinberg School of Medicine, Abbott Hall Suite 1004, 710 North Lake Shore Drive, Chicago, IL 60611, USA
* Corresponding author.
E-mail address: lbuenav1@jhmi.edu

Sleep Med Clin 14 (2019) 275–281
https://doi.org/10.1016/j.jsmc.2019.01.008
1556-407X/19/© 2019 Elsevier Inc. All rights reserved.

real world. It discusses 3 main issues. First, where and how should CBT-I be delivered and who should deliver it? Second, who is an appropriate candidate for CBT-I? Third, how does one measure quality care with CBT-I?

ISSUE 1: DELIVERY CONSIDERATIONS

Typically, insomnia treatment begins in primary care and is limited to pharmacotherapy and/or basic sleep hygiene education.[9,10] In some cases, insomnia treatment might be initiated in a mental health clinic. Again, the initial treatment is likely pharmacotherapy and/or sleep hygiene but might include CBT-I if there is a provider who is trained in behavioral sleep medicine. Although there are multiple reasons, Koffel and colleagues (2018) identified three general factors that make it difficult to deliver CBT-I in routine healthcare settings: (1) system barriers; (2) patient barriers; and (3) a lack of knowledge about and experience treating sleep disorders among most primary care providers.[11] Moreover, it is often not practical to have a CBT-I specialist available to see insomnia patients in a primary care setting because of the unpredictable nature of the presenting complaint. As a result, CBT-I is typically delivered in a sleep disorders clinic, mental health clinic, or other specialty clinic (ie, behavioral medicine).

Another controversial issue involves the training and credentials of the CBT-I provider. Typically, the provider is a licensed clinician who has specialized training in behavioral sleep medicine. However, there is disagreement about the level of training required. For example, is a doctoral degree (PhD, PsyD, or MD) required or is a master's degree with specialized training sufficient? This debate has carried over to the board certification for behavioral sleep medicine in which the decision to include master's level clinicians has been inconsistent. The current Diplomat of Behavioral Sleep Medicine allows for both master's and doctoral level providers. Among the driving forces for favoring a more inclusive approach is to increase the potential pool of providers. Currently, most CBT-I providers are concentrated in major metropolitan areas and are often affiliated with academic medical centers. There are relatively fewer CBT-I providers in community-based sleep clinics and a dearth of CBT-I providers in rural areas. The limited availability of trained CBT-I providers limits the practical delivery of CBT-I. Given these constraints, a major push in the dissemination of CBT-I has been to use alternate forms of delivery beyond traditional face-to-face individual therapy. The following sections review the research on the various forms of delivery.

Group Cognitive Behavioral Therapy for Insomnia

Group therapy is an example of a treatment delivery method in which CBT-I can be administered to reach a larger number of persons than traditional individual psychotherapy. In the only meta-analysis of randomized clinical trials (RCTs) for group-administered CBT-I, Koffel and colleagues[12] (2015) found 8 studies examining the efficacy of CBT-I administered in this format. Results demonstrated significant improvements in multiple outcome variables, including initial sleep onset, time spent awake during the night, sleep efficiency (SE), and total sleep time. Effect sizes ranged considerably by variable: from 1.13 to .29. Post-treatment treatment gains were observed at follow-up with small to large effect sizes (.29–.89), suggesting that group-administered CBT-I is effective and the benefits are largely maintained at follow-up. Advantages of choosing group therapy include the built-in social support aspect of the treatment, as well as fewer demands placed on the therapist to treat a larger volume of patients.[12] Although this format can be more efficient than individual therapy, it does not resolve the issue of reaching patients who live in rural areas or who cannot travel to the location that is offering group CBT-I. Koffel and colleagues[12] (2015) also reported that 2 of the 3 studies that compared group-administered CBT-I to individually administered CBT-I found that individual treatment was more effective, whereas the third study did not.

Telephone Cognitive Behavioral Therapy for Insomnia

To enhance access with fewer restrictions due to distance, CBT-I has been delivered via telephone and been shown to offer some advantages over traditional, in-person, 1-on-1 therapy. In 1 of the few RCTs examining telephone-delivered CBT-I, Arnedt and colleagues[13] (2013) argue that telephone-delivered CBT-I offers a low intensity, self-administered version of CBT-I that would be more effective than a minimal intervention, such as an information pamphlet. In their study, 4 CBT-I treatment modules were delivered over a 4 to 8 week period and compared with written CBT-I instructions. Individuals receiving telephone CBT-I demonstrated larger effect sizes (Cohen's d: 0.8–2.5) and a higher percentage of individuals were considered treatment responders based on predetermined criteria when compared with those receiving written instructions. Treatment gains were maintained at 12-week follow-up. Telephone-based interventions offer both advantages and disadvantages. They are readily accessible, cost-efficient, and allow for human interaction, including a therapeutic alliance. However, published RCTs studying the efficacy of telephone-based CBT-I are lacking. Consequently, there are no published standardized guidelines describing the structure and format of telephone delivery of CBT-I. Another practical concern pertains to health provider reimbursement. Outside the context of a research study, it is difficult to find telephone-based CBT-I because in many states telephone contact for nonphysician health care providers is not a covered service. Finally, face-to-face CBT-I treatments of at least 4 sessions in duration have been demonstrated to be superior to self-help interventions.[14]

Internet Cognitive Behavioral Therapy for Insomnia

Internet delivered CBT-I has and will continue to reach a large number of individuals struggling with insomnia; research supporting this delivery mechanism has grown significantly in the past 15 to 20 years.[15–17] In 1 systematic review of the literature, Zachariae and colleagues[17] (2016) found online CBT-I to improve insomnia severity, SE, subjective sleep quality, wake after sleep onset (WASO), sleep duration, and nocturnal awakenings (effect sizes range 0.21–1.09). Similarly, Seyffert and colleagues[15] (2016) also performed a systematic review and meta-analysis and found online CBT-I to produce improvements in SE, sleep duration, and insomnia severity with durable treatment effects observed 4 to 48 weeks post-treatment. In another meta-analysis of randomized controlled trials, Ye and colleagues[16] (2016) found improvements in sleep onset latency, WASO, sleep duration, SE, nocturnal awakenings, and insomnia severity. Online delivery of CBT-I offers several advantages compared with traditional in-person therapy. Namely, Internet-based CBT-I is highly structured, content-specific, cost-efficient (compared with traditional in-person therapy), and can provide a flexible therapeutic approach. Some of the concerns with Internet-based therapy pertain to the validity of online diagnoses. This is more apparent for medically complex patients. Patients with psychiatric comorbidities and/or whose sleep disturbance may be due to a sleep disorder other than insomnia should be referred to existing face-to-face services. There are also practical concerns. Although CBT is covered under some health insurance plans, it is not clear whether Internet-based CBT-I is covered. Finally, as previously mentioned, the available evidence indicates that any contact with a clinician may improve outcomes. With regard to CBT-I, specifically,

face-to-face treatments of at least 4 treatment sessions are more effective than self-help treatments.[14] Future research in this area should investigate (1) the characteristics of those patients likely to benefit from Internet-based interventions, (2) how to best integrate Internet interventions with existing services, and (3) optimal strategies for combining Internet interventions with pharmacotherapy.

With the availability of different CBT-I delivery options, there exist greater opportunities for innovation in implementing CBT-I. One example involves a stepped-care approach championed by Espie[18] (2009), who proposed a model to efficiently use resources at an earlier stage (eg, Internet or telephone delivery of CBT-I) and implement more intensive resources (eg, individual therapy with certified behavioral sleep specialist) as needed at later stages. Given that primary care is the typical entry point for people with insomnia, other efforts have been directed at integrating CBT-I into primary care clinics. This includes offering Internet-based CBT-I (as opposed to pharmacotherapy) for patients who complain of insomnia, or having nurse practitioners or physicians' assistants trained to deliver a more limited version of CBT-I (eg, brief behavior therapy for insomnia[19]). Finally, some recommendations are aimed at addressing patient-level factors. For example, Koffel and colleagues[11] (2018) found that lack of knowledge about CBT-I was among the first barriers for individuals deciding to seek treatment. Many people are unaware that a nonpharmacological treatment option exists and that CBT-I is effective.[20] In addition, many laypersons confuse sleep hygiene guidelines with CBT-I and mistakenly conclude that they have tried these strategies to change their habits, usually without benefit. Furthermore, accessibility-related barriers, such as long travel distances and long wait times to obtain an appointment with a specialty provider, are barriers that could be overcome with telemedicine or Internet-based delivery. Moreover, providing education to patients about CBT-I and providing resources to primary care clinics on alternate methods of delivering CBT-I could help address some of these patient-level barriers and increase utilization of CBT-I.

ISSUE 2: PATIENT CHARACTERISTICS

The previous sections illustrate the success researchers have had with expanding methods of treatment delivery. Although not as robust, researchers have attempted to determine factors contributing to treatment success across the spectrum of delivery mechanisms. The nature of

CBT-I is such that individuals with certain comorbid conditions are not likely to be suitable candidates (**Table 1**). CBT-I may pose some degree of risk for patients with excessive daytime sleepiness (EDS), or with bipolar or seizure disorder. Specifically, sleep deprivation, resulting from sleep restriction, lowers seizure threshold[21] and may trigger manic episodes[22] in vulnerable individuals. Sleep deprivation may also exacerbate parasomnias related to nonrapid eye movement (NREM) sleep transitions (eg, sleep walking, night terrors)[23,24] and exacerbate EDS to the point at which sleepiness may pose a safety risk with regard to operating a motor vehicle or heavy machinery, or impair judgment. Consequently, sleep restriction should be administered cautiously and conservatively with these populations. Patients should be closely monitored and safeguards put in place. Another documented collateral effect of CBT-I is paradoxic relaxation-induced anxiety,[25] which has been reported in approximately 15% of persons who attempt to practice relaxation. Patients with nocturnal panic attacks, which occur primarily during NREM sleep,[26] may be particularly susceptible because they seem to be more fearful of states that involve a lessening of conscious awareness.[27] However, these adverse events can be managed clinically.

Generally, little is known about rates of adherence and factors associated with patients' adherence to CBT-I. Typically, treatment success is often contingent or proportional to the amount of treatment completed. Studies investigating CBT-I rarely include adherence information and, when reported, the information is typically limited to the average number of sessions attended or overall study attrition. Objective measures of adherence are rarely used. Instead, self-report, particularly sleep diary data, is relied on for aspects of CBT-I for which it is more difficult to assess treatment adherence. Current data suggest that approximately 14% to 40% of research participants drop out of individual or group CBT-I before midtreatment.[28] A systematic review of CBT-I treatment adherence found that demographic (eg, age, gender, education), medical, and psychological variables are not consistently related to treatment adherence.[29] However, some studies have found that higher levels of pretreatment depression[30,31] and anxiety[32] have an association with poor adherence. Attitudes toward treatment, including motivation to change sleep behaviors,[33] higher treatment expectations,[34] greater self-efficacy,[35] and greater satisfaction with CBT-I,[36] were associated with better outcomes. Ong and colleagues[28] (2008) reported that short sleep duration and depressive symptoms were associated with premature withdrawal from group CBT-I. Possible barriers to treatment have also been discussed in relation to treatment adherence. One of the largest barriers relates specifically to implementation of sleep restriction therapy. Poor sleep quality ratings before treatment,[33] as well as how quickly sleep improves during treatment,[30,32,37] have been found to predict adherence. Severity of initial insomnia symptoms is thought to be an indicator of ultimate outcome but these results have also been inconsistent.[38,39] The methods to assess treatment adherence varied dramatically across studies, with little objectivity; in addition, there were no overall significantly reliable predictors of treatment adherence and

Table 1
Cognitive behavioral therapy for insomnia contraindications

Condition	CBT-I Technique	Mechanism	Consequences
Excessive Daytime Somnolence	Sleep restriction	Sleep deprivation	Impaired ability to operate motor vehicle or heavy equipment Impaired judgment that may affect patient safety or safety of others
Bipolar Disorder	Sleep restriction	Sleep deprivation	May trigger manic episode
Seizure Disorder	Sleep restriction	Sleep deprivation	May lower seizure threshold
Nonrapid Eye Movement Parasomnias (eg, sleep walking, night terrors)	Sleep restriction	Sleep deprivation	May exacerbate parasomnias
Nocturnal Panic Attacks	Relaxation training	Fear or anxiety triggered by psychological states associated with decreases in conscious awareness	Paradoxic relaxation-induced anxiety

success.[29] The authors advocate for objective measures of treatment adherence, including spouse reporting and actigraphy.

Prior psychological research has measured patient variables in psychotherapy to identify patient factors that affect psychotherapy treatment outcomes[40] and, sometimes specifically, outcomes for cognitive behavioral therapy. There are several challenges inherent in this area of research. Specifically, the wide range of variables investigated and the high degree of variability in measurement approaches, including research design, the heterogeneity of research participants studied, differences in therapist skill level and training, and the variability in clinical settings, make it difficult to arrive at valid conclusions about a set of specific patient variables that predict successful psychotherapy outcomes.

Determining the ideal candidate for CBT-I is likely to depend on a combination of situational factors, comorbid factors, and individual patient characteristics. The complexity of this situation makes predicting treatment success difficult. Motivation to change behavior is an additional patient characteristic that has drawn less intention. Because CBT-I requires an enormous amount of effort, it would seem to be beneficial to assess level of motivation. Seminal work in this area has examined motivation to change among several patient groups contemplating making a commitment to a course of treatment.[41] Research on the transtheoretical model has failed to predict a profile of successful behavior change, however. This is not particularly surprising given the complex combination of factors already implicated in successful implementation of CBT-I.

Overall, a limited number of studies have used an explicit theoretic model to examine adherence to CBT-I. Hebert and colleagues[42] (2010) used the theory of planned behavior[43] in combination with the transtheoretical model of behavior change in an effort to maximize treatment adherence. Results, however, suggested that neither theory significantly helped predict attrition. Bouchard and colleagues[35] (2003) hypothesized that self-efficacy, a concept derived from social cognitive theory, may be useful in predicting adherence to CBT-I, whereas Vincent and Hameed[32] (2003) theorized that the health beliefs model may help explain nonadherence to CBT-I.

ISSUE 3: MEASURING QUALITY CARE

Another major challenge involving implementation of CBT-I is measuring quality of care for people with insomnia. In the United States, health care policies are shifting toward quality reporting as an incentive for reimbursement of services. To promote high-quality, patient-centered care, the American Academy of Sleep Medicine commissioned a task force to develop quality measures.[44] Recommendations for insomnia included 4 process measures (assessment of sleep quality, delivery of evidence-based treatment, assessment of daytime functioning, assessment of adverse effects) and 2 outcome measures (improvement of sleep, improvement of daytime functioning).[45] The outcome measures represent the desired improvements or benefits achieved with the service and the process measures represent the steps taken to achieve the outcomes. Assessment of both process and outcome measures thus provides an indication of the quality of care being delivered for people with insomnia at a particular clinical site. Implementation of these process and outcome measures (eg, audit of electronic medical records) would provide a standard methodology for determining if a particular clinic was delivering quality care for patients with insomnia, which could be used for reimbursement purposes or as part of a self-study for improvement of patient services.

Although these quality measures provide a starting point, they raise several issues with regard to implementation. As noted previously, insomnia treatments occur across many different types of clinical settings, which makes it difficult to implement standard assessments. For example, systematic assessment of daytime functioning and adverse effects could be more difficult in a primary care setting compared with a specialty sleep clinic due to the variations in presenting complaint and patient flow noted previously. Further complicating matters is the increase of Internet-based delivery of CBT-I. Currently, Internet-based delivery is considered outside of the health care system so it is unclear if and how quality measures would be applied to an automated program. In addition, given the patient-level factors described previously, it can be argued that quality of care could come from a direct-to-consumer approach. For example, informing patients about treatment options for insomnia and educating patients about the benefits of CBT-I versus sleep hygiene could enable patients to become more proactive in seeking CBT-I or in discussing this as a preferred treatment option with their health care provider.

SUMMARY AND DIRECTIONS FOR FUTURE RESEARCH

With CBT-I, there is now an established treatment of insomnia. As highlighted in this article, much work remains in understanding contextual factors related to the delivery of CBT-I in the real world. With the increase in scalable forms of delivery using telemedicine and Internet-based programs,

CBT-I no longer is limited by a shortage of qualified providers or by the remoteness of a geographic location but instead by new questions regarding oversight and regulation of these programs. There remains very little known about which patient characteristics predict treatment success and adherence to treatment, or who is likely to experience adverse events. Further research in this area could determine for whom CBT-I is recommended or for whom an alternative treatment might be warranted. Finally, the development and implementation of quality measures can be a valuable tool in assessing the extent to which CBT-I is being implemented in the clinical setting and the extent to which patients are benefitting from CBT-I in the real world. These issues point to the need for further research in implementation science that can help identify and remove barriers for the delivery of CBT-I in the real world.

REFERENCES

1. Qaseem A, Kansagara D, Forciea MA, et al, Clinical Guidelines Committee of the American College of Physicians. Management of chronic insomnia disorder in adults: a clinical practice guideline from the American College of Physicians. Ann Intern Med 2016;165(2):125–33.
2. Riemann D, Baglioni C, Bassetti C, et al. European guideline for the diagnosis and treatment of insomnia. J Sleep Res 2017;26(6):675–700.
3. Schutte-Rodin S, Broch L, Buysse D, et al. Clinical guideline for the evaluation and management of chronic insomnia in adults. J Clin Sleep Med 2008;4(5):487–504.
4. Conley S, Redeker NS. Cognitive behavioral therapy for insomnia in the context of cardiovascular conditions. Curr Sleep Med Rep 2015;1(3):157–65.
5. Smith MT, Finan PH, Buenaver LF, et al. Cognitive-behavioral therapy for insomnia in knee osteoarthritis: a randomized, double-blind, active placebo-controlled clinical trial. Arthritis Rheumatol 2015;67(5):1221–33.
6. Talbot LS, Maguen S, Metzler TJ, et al. Cognitive behavioral therapy for insomnia in posttraumatic stress disorder: a randomized controlled trial. Sleep 2014;37(2):327–41.
7. Bei B, Asarnow LD, Krystal A, et al. Treating insomnia in depression: insomnia related factors predict long-term depression trajectories. J Consult Clin Psychol 2018;86(3):282–93.
8. Myers E, Startup H, Freeman D. Cognitive behavioural treatment of insomnia in individuals with persistent persecutory delusions: a pilot trial. J Behav Ther Exp Psychiatry 2011;42(3):330–6.
9. Everitt H, McDermott L, Leydon G, et al. GPs' management strategies for patients with insomnia: a survey and qualitative interview study. Br J Gen Pract 2014;64(619):e112–9.
10. Cheung JM, Atternas K, Melchior M, et al. Primary health care practitioner perspectives on the management of insomnia: a pilot study. Aust J Prim Health 2014;20(1):103–12.
11. Koffel E, Bramoweth AD, Ulmer CS. Increasing access to and utilization of cognitive behavioral therapy for insomnia (CBT-I): a narrative review. J Gen Intern Med 2018;33(6):955–62.
12. Koffel EA, Koffel JB, Gehrman PR. A meta-analysis of group cognitive behavioral therapy for insomnia. Sleep Med Rev 2015;19:6–16.
13. Arnedt JT, Cuddihy L, Swanson LM, et al. Randomized controlled trial of telephone-delivered cognitive behavioral therapy for chronic insomnia. Sleep 2013;36(3):353–62.
14. van Straten A, van der Zweerde T, Kleiboer A, et al. Cognitive and behavioral therapies in the treatment of insomnia: a meta-analysis. Sleep Med Rev 2018;38:3–16.
15. Seyffert M, Lagisetty P, Landgraf J, et al. Internet-delivered cognitive behavioral therapy to treat insomnia: a systematic review and meta-analysis. PLoS One 2016;11(2):e0149139.
16. Ye YY, Chen NK, Chen J, et al. Internet-based cognitive-behavioural therapy for insomnia (ICBT-i): a meta-analysis of randomised controlled trials. BMJ Open 2016;6(11):e010707.
17. Zachariae R, Lyby MS, Ritterband LM, et al. Efficacy of internet-delivered cognitive-behavioral therapy for insomnia - a systematic review and meta-analysis of randomized controlled trials. Sleep Med Rev 2016;30:1–10.
18. Espie CA. "Stepped care": a health technology solution for delivering cognitive behavioral therapy as a first line insomnia treatment. Sleep 2009;32(12):1549–58.
19. Troxel WM, Germain A, Buysse DJ. Clinical management of insomnia with brief behavioral treatment (BBTI). Behav Sleep Med 2012;10(4):266–79.
20. Stinson K, Tang NK, Harvey AG. Barriers to treatment seeking in primary insomnia in the United Kingdom: a cross-sectional perspective. Sleep 2006;29(12):1643–6.
21. Fountain NB, Kim JS, Lee SI. Sleep deprivation activates epileptiform discharges independent of the activating effects of sleep. J Clin Neurophysiol 1998;15(1):69–75.
22. Colombo C, Benedetti F, Barbini B, et al. Rate of switch from depression into mania after therapeutic sleep deprivation in bipolar depression. Psychiatry Res 1999;86(3):267–70.
23. Mahowald MW, Bornemann MC, Schenck CH. Parasomnias. Semin Neurol 2004;24(3):283–92.
24. Mahowald MW, Schenck CH. NREM sleep parasomnias. Neurol Clin 1996;14(4):675–96.

25. Heide FJ, Borkovec TD. Relaxation-induced anxiety: paradoxical anxiety enhancement due to relaxation training. J Consult Clin Psychol 1983;51(2):171–82.

26. Mellman TA, Uhde TW. Electroencephalographic sleep in panic disorder. A focus on sleep-related panic attacks. Arch Gen Psychiatry 1989;46(2):178–84.

27. Craske MG, Lang AJ, Tsao JC, et al. Reactivity to interoceptive cues in nocturnal panic. J Behav Ther Exp Psychiatry 2001;32(3):173–90.

28. Ong JC, Kuo TF, Manber R. Who is at risk for dropout from group cognitive-behavior therapy for insomnia? J Psychosom Res 2008;64(4):419–25.

29. Matthews EE, Arnedt JT, McCarthy MS, et al. Adherence to cognitive behavioral therapy for insomnia: a systematic review. Sleep Med Rev 2013;17(6):453–64.

30. McChargue DE, Sankaranarayanan J, Visovsky CG, et al. Predictors of adherence to a behavioral therapy sleep intervention during breast cancer chemotherapy. Support Care Cancer 2012;20(2):245–52.

31. Manber R, Bernert RA, Suh S, et al. CBT for insomnia in patients with high and low depressive symptom severity: adherence and clinical outcomes. J Clin Sleep Med 2011;7(6):645–52.

32. Vincent NK, Hameed H. Relation between adherence and outcome in the group treatment of insomnia. Behav Sleep Med 2003;1(3):125–39.

33. Matthews EE, Schmiege SJ, Cook PF, et al. Adherence to cognitive behavioral therapy for insomnia (CBTI) among women following primary breast cancer treatment: a pilot study. Behav Sleep Med 2012;10(3):217–29.

34. Tremblay V, Savard J, Ivers H. Predictors of the effect of cognitive behavioral therapy for chronic insomnia comorbid with breast cancer. J Consult Clin Psychol 2009;77(4):742–50.

35. Bouchard S, Bastien C, Morin CM. Self-efficacy and adherence to cognitive-behavioral treatment of insomnia. Behav Sleep Med 2003;1(4):187–99.

36. Chambers MJ, Alexander SD. Assessment and prediction of outcome for a brief behavioral insomnia treatment program. J Behav Ther Exp Psychiatry 1992;23(4):289–97.

37. Harvey L, Inglis SJ, Espie CA. Insomniacs' reported use of CBT components and relationship to long-term clinical outcome. Behav Res Ther 2002;40(1):75–83.

38. Perlis M, Aloia M, Millikan A, et al. Behavioral treatment of insomnia: a clinical case series study. J Behav Med 2000;23(2):149–61.

39. Morgan K, Dixon S, Mathers N, et al. Psychological treatment for insomnia in the management of long-term hypnotic drug use: a pragmatic randomised controlled trial. Br J Gen Pract 2003;53(497):923–8.

40. Garfield SL. Research on client variables in psychotherapy. In: Bergin AE, Garfield SL, editors. Handbook of psychotherapy and behavior change. 4th edition. Oxford (England): John Wiley & Sons; 1994. p. 190–228.

41. Prochaska JO, DiClemente CC. Stages and processes of self-change of smoking: toward an integrative model of change. J Consult Clin Psychol 1983;51(3):390–5.

42. Hebert EA, Vincent N, Lewycky S, et al. Attrition and adherence in the online treatment of chronic insomnia. Behav Sleep Med 2010;8(3):141–50.

43. Ajzen I, Madden TJ. Prediction of goal-directed behavior: attitudes, intentions, and perceived behavioral control. J Exp Soc Psychol 1986;22(5):453–74.

44. Morgenthaler TI, Aronsky AJ, Carden KA, et al. Measurement of quality to improve care in sleep medicine. J Clin Sleep Med 2015;11(3):279–91.

45. Edinger JD, Buysse DJ, Deriy L, et al. Quality measures for the care of patients with insomnia. J Clin Sleep Med 2015;11(3):311–34.

Online Delivery of Cognitive Behavioral Therapy-Insomnia
Considerations and Controversies

Michelle L. Drerup, PsyD, DBSM[a],*,
Samina Ahmed-Jauregui, PsyD[b]

KEYWORDS

- Cognitive behavioral therapy for insomnia • Chronic insomnia • Internet • Online • Dissemination
- CBT-I

KEY POINTS

- Web-based interventions for insomnia have increased accessibility to cognitive behavioral therapy for insomnia (CBT-I).
- Research on the effectiveness of online CBT-I has grown exponentially over the past decade.
- Strengths of online CBT-I include increased convenience and accessibility to this treatment intervention.
- Challenges of online CBT-I include decreased tailoring of program and higher dropout rates.
- Future research needs to explore dissemination and implementation of online CBT-I in a stepped care model of insomnia treatment.

INTRODUCTION

Delivery of health care via the Internet has rapidly evolved and expanded over the past decade and web and mobile technology are here to stay. Internet interventions have been developed for various psychological conditions that have a strong behavioral component, including depression, various anxiety disorders, and chronic insomnia.

Chronic insomnia is a major public health concern, and the burden of insomnia on both the individual and society is considerable. The efficacy of in-person cognitive behavioral therapy for insomnia (CBT-I) has been robustly researched and supported among individuals ranging in age from childhood to elderly adults, as well as more complex insomnia with comorbid medical and psychiatric conditions.[1–6] Despite being highly effective, individual CBT-I has been criticized as being expensive and time consuming. Perhaps the most valid concern has been a lack of availability and access to CBT-I as the population that suffers from insomnia largely surpasses the number of trained providers.

Numerous efforts and advancements have been made in the past decade to provide a broader and more rapid dissemination of CBT-I treatment, some of which have already been discussed in earlier articles. The focus of this article is to review the most recent literature on the efficacy as well as strengths and limitations of online delivery of CBT-I, exploring various considerations (**Box 1**) and controversies that exist in this relatively new yet burgeoning area of behavioral sleep medicine (BSM).

Disclosure Statement: No disclosures.
[a] Sleep Disorders Center, Cleveland Clinic, Cleveland Clinic Lerner College of Medicine, 9500 Euclid Avenue, S73, Cleveland, OH 44195, USA; [b] Department of Pulmonology and Sleep Medicine, University Hospitals, 11100 Euclid Avenue, Cleveland, OH 44106, USA
* Corresponding author.
E-mail address: drerupm@ccf.org

Sleep Med Clin 14 (2019) 283–290
https://doi.org/10.1016/j.jsmc.2019.02.001

Box 1
Practice points

- Consider potential consequences of fully automated, unguided online treatment with specific consideration for attrition and lack of therapist support.
- Identify patient factors that promote and hinder use of online treatment.
  - Environmental factors: access to Internet, experience with technology, proximity to behavioral sleep medicine provider, and demographic considerations (ie, age, sex, and race).
  - Physical health factors: mobility difficulties, medication side effects, chronic pain and fatigue, and untreated sleep disorders.
  - Mental health factors: depressed mood, anxiety, cognitive function, and substance use.
- Consider addition of medication tapering plan that coincides with online CBT-I program.

EFFECTIVENESS OF ONLINE COGNITIVE BEHAVIORAL THERAPY-INSOMNIA

The empirical basis of CBT-I as the first-line treatment for insomnia was established with in-person, individual delivery of treatment by a trained therapist. Subsequently, the efficacy of online CBT-I in improving sleep difficulties is also well established in the literature. The research studies can be separated into guided and unguided delivery of online CBT-I. Guided online CBT-I is defined as an automated program combined with therapeutic support usually delivered via email or chat function in the program. Research shows that guided CBT-I programs have been effective in improving sleep quality and daytime fatigue and reducing overall severity of insomnia in comparison with nontreatment control groups.[7,8] One study also found that providing support in the form of weekly emails accompanying an online CBT-I program enhances the benefits of internet-delivered treatment for insomnia on several variables including sleep measures, insomnia severity, depression, and anxiety.[9] An overview of additional randomized controlled trials (RCT) including those discussed can be found in 3 recently published meta-analyses.[10–12]

In contrast, fully automated or unguided online CBT-I does not include therapeutic support. For example, one RCT compared a 6-session online CBT-I program with a 6-session online Image Rehearsal Therapy program as placebo and a

treatment as usual condition.[13] The online treatment conditions were delivered by an animated personal therapist, with automated web and email support. Results indicated superior improvement in sleep parameters and insomnia symptoms for the CBT-I condition as compared with the placebo and treatment as usual conditions. Two other fully automated programs also demonstrated effectiveness in improving sleep-onset latency, wake after sleep onset, sleep efficiency, and insomnia severity.[14,15] The effect sizes of these RCTs are in a similar range as guided online CBT-I interventions.

One of the benefits of fully automated programs is that they do not require any clinician time and are likely the most cost-efficient service available. Notably, there is a growing body of research that has demonstrated that weekly therapist support as an adjunct to structured, web-based CBT for the treatment of depression and anxiety symptoms enhances treatment adherence and outcomes; programs without formal support have highly variable and typically lower completion and success rates.[16] Thus, additional studies of fully automated online CBT-I programs with long-term follow-up are needed to establish effectiveness in comparison to guided online CBT-I treatment.

Integration of BSM specialists within online CBT-I programs has been suggested as a way to facilitate patient engagement, monitor progress to decrease dropout, address any adverse events reported, problem-solve barriers, and respond to patient questions that may arise as the patient is completing the program.[17] Determining patient factors that help predict who might benefit from the additional support of a BSM specialist versus who might benefit from fully automated programs would also be an important step in enhancing efficacy while not limiting scalability and dissemination efforts. Numerous professional concerns arise with this potential role, including licensure laws (eg, providing services outside of state), competency, and scope of practice that need to be addressed before this becomes a viable option. The additional time and cost associated with a BSM expert guidance of online programs should be explored to see if this leads to increased adherence and improved outcomes to offset the additional costs. A related concern is that BSM clinicians may feel threatened and eventually render their services obsolete with the proliferation of automated online delivery of CBT-I. Given the large number of people in need of this treatment, this is not a likely outcome. Internet interventions should be regarded as a compliment to in-person services rather than as a replacement for in-person, face to face treatment, especially for more complex and severe insomnia.

COMPARISON TO IN-PERSON TREATMENT

Despite established effectiveness of online CBT-I, there is limited research comparing the effectiveness of online CBT-I with in-person delivery of treatment. One RCT compared the effectiveness of guided online and in-person CBT-I to a waitlist condition.[18] Results indicated superior performance of in-person treatment as compared with online treatment; however, results also suggested that online CBT-I treatment may offer a potentially cost-effective alternative to and complement in-person treatment. Similarly, in a sample of active duty military personnel, both in-person and unguided online CBT-I were significantly superior than the control group, which consisted of phone call assessments.[19] However, in-person treatment was better than online treatment on self-reported sleep quality and dysfunctional beliefs and attitudes about sleep. In another RCT with a sample of adolescents, guided online CBT-I therapy was found to be as effective as in-person group CBT-I therapy when compared with a waitlist condition.[20] These results were consistent in a Swedish sample of adults with comparable effect sizes when comparing guided online CBT-I with group CBT-I.[21] In comparison to telehealth delivery of CBT-I, online CBT-I produced equivalent changes in insomnia severity and was favored by patients over telehealth services.[22] Despite superior performance of in-person treatment in individual studies, meta-analyses data suggest effects of online CBT-I are in the range of conventional in-person treatment in regard to sleep parameters (eg, total sleep time, sleep onset, sleep efficiency, etc.).[12]

IMPACT OF ONLINE COGNITIVE BEHAVIORAL THERAPY-INSOMNIA ON COMORBID MENTAL AND PHYSICAL HEALTH

Insomnia is highly comorbid with other mental health conditions (eg, depression and anxiety) and mutually exacerbate clinical trajectories and treatment outcomes. Results on the effectiveness of online CBT-I in reducing depression symptoms have been demonstrated. One study found online CBT-I significantly improved mental health constructs such as depression, anxiety, quality of life, and fatigue as compared with a waitlist condition, producing large effect sizes.[23] Another study used a fully automated online CBT-I program and found that it was successful in reducing depressive symptoms (ie, PHQ-9 scores) as compared with a waitlist condition, but it did not prevent the onset of major depressive disorder.[24] A meta-analysis consisting of 10 RCTs was conducted to assess the effectiveness of online CBT-I in the

treatment of insomnia with comorbid depression and/or anxiety disorder.[25] Effect sizes for sleep parameters were found to be consistent with non-comorbid insomnia. Effect sizes for the treatment of comorbid depression and anxiety were small and suggested positive effects of online CBT-I on both comorbid disorders. Feasibility studies have also suggested that online CBT-I might be an effective treatment in patients with alcohol use disorder[26] and posttraumatic stress disorder.[27]

A recent meta-analysis also assessed for efficacy of treatment across a range of demographic groups.[28] The online CBT-I condition yielded greater reductions in both insomnia and depression severity than the control group, which were maintained at follow-up. Demographic variables (ie, income, race, sex, age, and education) were not significant moderators of the treatment effects, suggesting that online CBT-I is comparably efficacious across a wide range of demographic groups. Furthermore, differences in attrition were found based on SES, but attrition did not differ between white and black participants. These results demonstrate the potential role of online CBT-I in treating insomnia and comorbid depression in a demographically diverse population.

Another meta-analysis reported small to medium positive effect across comorbid outcomes, with larger effects on psychiatric conditions compared with medical conditions.[6] Notably, the impact of online CBT-I on physical health has been less widely studied despite the relatively high comorbidity between insomnia and other physical health conditions. RCTs suggest that online CBT-I can be used effectively to treat insomnia in patients with physical health conditions such as elevated blood pressure[29] and Parkinson disease[30] and has also been found to be effective in reducing physical health complaints such as tinnitus.[31,32] In a sample of women diagnosed with chronic migraines and insomnia, results supported feasibility and acceptability of online CBT-I, with large effects on reducing insomnia and small effects on reducing headache disability.[33] In contrast, patients who endorsed no pain, mild pain, or moderate/severe pain were found to have equivalent pre- to posttreatment improvements in insomnia severity and sleep parameters; however, improvement in pain complaints was not noted.[34]

A recent RCT implemented online CBT-I in a large sample of Danish breast cancer survivors.[35] Effect sizes ranged small to large for all sleep-related outcomes including fatigue, and improvement was maintained at 15-week postintervention. These findings were consistent with a previous, pilot study.[36] Online CBT-I seems to be effective in breast cancer survivors, with additional benefit in terms of reduced fatigue. This low-cost treatment could be incorporated in cancer rehabilitation and other physical rehabilitation programs. Additional studies evaluating the impact of online CBT-I on physical health concerns such as fatigue syndromes and chronic pain is warranted.

COST-EFFECTIVENESS OF ONLINE COGNITIVE BEHAVIORAL THERAPY-INSOMNIA

One restrictive factor of wider dissemination of online CBT-I is cost. One of the advantages that is often cited is that online CBT-I is less expensive than in-person treatment and a more cost-effective way to deliver treatment. However, one must ask the question who is bearing the cost of this treatment? Initial upfront costs for the development of an online CBT-I program and secure online systems to provide the program are often not taken into account. In addition, time and resources spent responding to queries/emails from users is also often unaccounted for expense. Arguably the biggest financial concern is that unfortunately, to the authors' awareness, few, if any, insurance providers in the United States cover online CBT-I as a benefit or provide reimbursement for cost of programs. Costs vary significantly among different online CBT-I programs and depending on an individual's insurance coverage and copay per session, in-person CBT-I may be less expensive for some individuals. Examining the impact of implementing online CBT-I on health care costs is likely an important step in seeking reimbursement from insurance companies.

Because of the extent that insomnia may affect productivity and health care costs, employee wellness programs should also consider offering reimbursement or incentives to employees for using an online CBT-I program. For example, one study conducted in a Fortune 500 company found a reduction in cost by effects of online CBT-I on presenteeism, but effects on absenteeism were not significant.[37] Similar results were found in an RCT of teachers endorsing significant work-related stress, with a cost saving of US$512 per participant.[38] The reduction in costs was mainly driven by the effects of the intervention on presenteeism and to a lesser degree by reduced absenteeism. Thus, online CBT-I can potentially reduce work-related costs, specifically work productivity and impairment; future research studies on the cost/benefits of online CBT-I are needed. The protocol of a current active study investigating feasibility, cost-effectiveness, and cost-utility of a guided online CBT-I intervention for patients who seek treatment from their general practitioner has been published.[39]

MEDIATORS AND MODERATORS OF ONLINE COGNITIVE BEHAVIORAL THERAPY-INSOMNIA EFFICACY

Although efficacy of online CBT-I is established, mediators and moderators of effects remain undetermined. Identification of modifiable mechanisms by which the treatment works may guide efforts to further improve the efficacy of online insomnia treatment. Emphasis on cognitive therapy and addressing sleep-related cognitions has been identified as a mediating factor. One RCT assessed how attributional, cognitive, and psychopathological symptoms may mediate sleep improvement.[40] Results indicated online CBT-I treatment modified sleep-related attributions, night-time thought content, and psychopathology symptoms (eg, depressed mood, anxiety, and stress) and was found to partly mediate improvement in DSM-5–defined insomnia symptoms. A second RCT compared online CBT-I with a waitlist condition and found dysfunctional beliefs and safety behaviors mediated the effects of treatment on insomnia severity and sleep efficiency.[41]

Adherence to treatment is also commonly identified as a modifying factor of treatment efficacy. Studies suggest that guidance of treatment further improves treatment outcomes such as weekly email reminders[9] and weekly phone check-in.[42] Online CBT-I seems to be a better fit for self-motivated individuals while others may benefit from the increased accountability that comes with in-person therapy. Lack of guidance and accountability may also be contributing to higher dropout rates. A recent meta-analysis reported the average dropout rate in online CBT-I was 24.7%.[11] Studies of traditional in-person individual and group CBT-I observed much lower dropout rates, ranging from 0% to 8%.[1–3] However, when looking outside of RCTs, dropout rates for in-person and group CBT-I in clinic settings ranged from 14% to 40%, which is more consistent with the dropout rates for online CBT-I.[43] Future research studies may benefit from focusing on what enhance effectiveness of guided online treatment by differentiating between factors such as better treatment adherence, greater accountability by the patient, working with a sleep "expert," and social support.

ONLINE COGNITIVE BEHAVIORAL THERAPY-INSOMNIA AS ENTRY LEVEL OF STEPPED CARE MODEL FOR INSOMNIA

Online CBT-I has greatly expanded the scalability of this treatment enhancing the potential to reach a much wider audience than the traditional methods of delivery. As population health management gains momentum, several stepped care models for delivery of CBT-I have been proposed.[44–46] Stepped care models are typically conceptualized as a pyramid with the primary goal of managing large patient volumes using lower treatment approaches. Online CBT-I has been recommended as an entry-level intervention, or the base of the pyramid, with individuals "stepping up" to more advanced and intensive CBT-I delivery methods, based on response to treatment (**Fig. 1**).

As one moves up the tiers of the pyramid, the type of service or delivery model involves more resources, increased expertise, and more individualization of the treatment, culminating with individually tailored CBT-I delivered by a BSM expert. Online CBT-I and other self-help tools are the most accessible and will likely manage the highest volume of the population. One assumption of stepped care models is that patients will move up to a higher level or intensity of care if they did not benefit from a lower tier intervention. However, numerous implementation concerns arise including the following:

- Patients often equate CBT-I to sleep hygiene and may not attempt online CBT-I.
- Patients may become frustrated if not benefiting from online CBT-I and dropout of treatment if they do not have more individualized guidance/plans.
- Patients may equate all CBT-I delivery methods as equal and be unaware that additional more intensive services are available.

Ideally, individuals using online CBT-I would be assessed and referred for use of the program by a health care provider who is skilled at differential diagnosis of basic sleep disorders. This provider will continue to observe the referred patient during and after completion of the program to assess for treatment response, barriers to treatment, and successful termination of treatment and next steps of care. However, to increase access and availability of care, "self-help" strategies including many of the online programs are available to all comers and not necessarily followed by a provider. There is concern that if people are not adequately screened or assessed for other issues that may be contributing to their sleep difficulties, not only will they potentially not benefit from CBT-I but also will not necessarily address the other medical/psychiatric condition that might be affecting sleep. Implementation of stepped care works best when a "patient navigator" monitors progress (or lack thereof) and symptom, problem-solves potential barriers to implementing

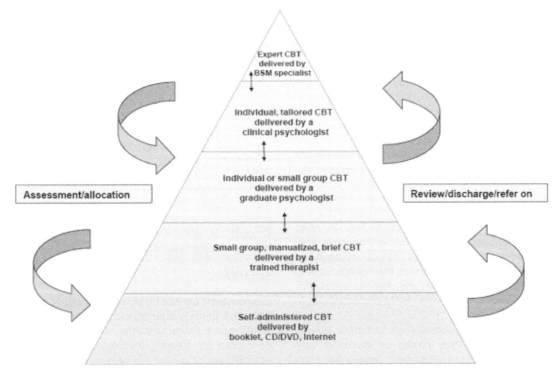

Fig. 1. A stepped care model for delivering cognitive behavioral therapy for insomnia. (*From* Espie CA. "Stepped care": a health technology solution for delivering cognitive behavioral therapy as a first line insomnia treatment. Sleep 2009;32(12):1554; with permission.)

treatment, and provides support as the patient completes the program. In addition, if a patient does not fully respond to the online intervention the patient navigator can assist in connecting patient to more intensive interventions until therapeutic goals are met.

Currently, online CBT-I does not modify specific treatment strategies to accommodate individuals whose insomnia is affected by another physical or mental health condition or sleep disorder such as obstructive sleep apnea. For instance, if a BSM expert was seeing a patient for in-person CBT-I who had insomnia comorbid with multiple sclerosis, the clinician could potentially tailor the plan based on the individual's disease state, which might include accounting for limitations in mobility that might impede implementation of stimulus control, as well as fatigue levels that may make avoidance of napping problematic for the patient. This further supports the importance of identifying factors and traits that may help us predict who is a better candidate for online CBT-I and who would benefit from in-person treatment.

As the stepped care model of insomnia indicates, increased access to CBT-I is arguably one of the major strengths of Internet delivery of this intervention. Currently, most CBT-I providers practice in large metropolitan areas in the United States, with 58% residing in just 12 states.[47] Many people may not have access to CBT-I due to lack of providers in their geographic area. Online CBT-I provides access to individuals who live in rural or remote areas or in states with limited provider access to a treatment that would otherwise be unavailable to them. Online CBT-I also provides an option for those with limited mobility due to other health conditions or difficulty obtaining transportation to health care appointments.

Regarding technology, 2018 estimates suggest that approximately 9 out of 10 Americans have access to the Internet, but roughly one-third of American adults do not have broadband Internet service at home. Reports have found that racial minorities, older adults, rural residents, and those with lower income and education levels are less likely to have broadband services at home, therefore, lacking the technology necessary to participate in online CBT-I effectively.[48] In fact, the individuals who lack access to technology are often the same population who lack access to BSM providers due to geographic area.

Future research should seek to further investigate a stepped-care model or insomnia care path. Specifically, how to best assess for entry level into the model and what factors may suggest more intense levels of treatment are warranted. Systems and processes need to be in place to

---

Box 2
Future research agenda

- Effectiveness of online CBT-I in a population with insomnia comorbid with other physical and mental health conditions.
- Exploration of mediators and moderators of online CBT-I outcomes.
- Role of online CBT-I in population health management of insomnia following a stepped care model.
- Benefits and cost-effectiveness of additional therapist guidance and support during use of online programs.
- Potential role and/or limits of online CBT-I in reducing use of sleep medication.

---

identify nonresponders to online treatment and provide delineated steps on how to proceed with more intensive and individualized services. Attention to accessibility and barriers to seeking treatment should also be considered.

TAPERING SLEEP MEDICATIONS

Another area that has not been extensively explored with online CBT-I is impact on decreasing or discontinuing use of sleep medication. On review, most of the existing online CBT-I programs do not specifically address sleep medication use or tapering in the intervention and no significant changes with sleep medication use was reported despite effectiveness of treatment.[7,13,14] The studies that have reported significantly lower use of sleep medication 1 to 3 years following intervention have been completed with a therapist-guided online CBT-I program in which medication use was specifically addressed.[49,50] Limited research has been done in this area to date and should be an area of focus for future research, especially to help guide the stepped care model of insomnia. Implementing a provider-approved medication tapering schedule to coincide with the online treatment protocol may be advantageous for the patient.

SUMMARY

Online CBT-I will not be able to replace in-person care, but there is little doubt that it will continue to grow as a powerful component of the stepped care plan for treating insomnia. Research has established that online CBT-I is an effective treatment of insomnia in the adult population, with improvements across a range of sleep measures (eg, sleep efficiency, sleep quality, wake after sleep onset, sleep onset latency, and total sleep time) and insomnia severity.[11] However, additional research is needed to address the current gaps in the literature such as comparison to in-person treatment, mediating and moderating factors of treatment effectiveness, adaptation of treatment with comorbid conditions, and consideration for medication discontinuation (**Box 2**). Most importantly, the field needs to emphasize scalability of treatment by conducting dissemination studies establishing CBT-I as the entry level intervention in a stepped care model of insomnia treatment in real-world clinical practice.

REFERENCES

1. Edinger JD, Wohlgemuth WK, Radtke RA, et al. Cognitive behavioral therapy for treatment of chronic primary insomnia: a randomized controlled trial. JAMA 2001;285(14):1856–64.
2. Morin CM, Colecchi C, Stone J, et al. Behavioral and pharmacological therapies for late-life insomnia: a randomized controlled trial. JAMA 1999;281(11):991–9.
3. Sivertsen B, Omvik S, Pallesen S, et al. Cognitive behavioral therapy vs zopiclone for treatment of chronic primary insomnia in older adults: a randomized controlled trial. JAMA 2006;295(24):2851–8.
4. Ma ZR, Shi LJ, Deng MH. Efficacy of cognitive behavioral therapy in children and adolescents with insomnia: a systematic review and meta-analysis. Braz J Med Biol Res 2018;51(6):e7070.
5. Trauer JM, Qian MY, Doyle JS, et al. Cognitive behavioral therapy for chronic insomnia: a systematic review and meta-analysis. Ann Intern Med 2015;163(3):191–204.
6. Wu JQ, Appleman ER, Salazar RD, et al. Cognitive Behavioral therapy for insomnia comorbid with psychiatric and medical conditions: a meta-analysis. JAMA Intern Med 2015;175(9):1461–72.
7. van Straten A, Emmelkamp J, de Wit J, et al. Guided Internet-delivered cognitive behavioural treatment for insomnia: a randomized trial. Psychol Med 2014;44(7):1521–32.
8. Anderson KN, Goldsmith P, Gardiner A. A pilot evaluation of an online cognitive behavioral therapy for insomnia disorder - targeted screening and interactive Web design lead to improved sleep in a community population. Nat Sci Sleep 2014;6:43–9.
9. Lancee J, van den Bout J, Sorbi MJ, et al. Motivational support provided via email improves the effectiveness of internet-delivered self-help treatment for insomnia: a randomized trial. Behav Res Ther 2013;51(12):797–805.
10. Ye YY, Chen NK, Chen J, et al. Internet-based cognitive-behavioural therapy for insomnia (ICBT-i): a meta-analysis of randomised controlled trials. BMJ Open 2016;6(11):e010707.
11. Zachariae R, Lyby MS, Ritterband LM, et al. Efficacy of internet-delivered cognitive-behavioral therapy for insomnia - a systematic review and meta-analysis of randomized controlled trials. Sleep Med Rev 2016; 30:1–10.
12. Seyffert M, Lagisetty P, Landgraf J, et al. Internet-delivered cognitive behavioral therapy to treat insomnia: a systematic review and meta-analysis. PLoS One 2016;11(2):e0149139.
13. Espie CA, Kyle SD, Williams C, et al. A randomized, placebo-controlled trial of online cognitive behavioral therapy for chronic insomnia disorder delivered via an automated media-rich web application. Sleep 2012;35(6):769–81.
14. Ritterband LM, Thorndike FP, Gonder-Frederick LA, et al. Efficacy of an Internet-based behavioral intervention for adults with insomnia. Arch Gen Psychiatry 2009;66(7):692–8.
15. Vincent N, Lewycky S. Logging on for better sleep: RCT of the effectiveness of online treatment for insomnia. Sleep 2009;32(6):807–15.
16. Spek V, Cuijpers P, Nyklícek I, et al. Internet-based cognitive behaviour therapy for symptoms of depression and anxiety: a meta-analysis. Psychol Med 2007;37(3):319–28.
17. Ong JC, Crawford MR. Understanding eCBT-I - knowing is half the battle. Sleep Med Rev 2016;30: 83–4.
18. Lancee J, van Straten A, Morina N, et al. Guided online or face-to-face cognitive behavioral treatment for insomnia: a randomized wait-list controlled trial. Sleep 2016;39(1):183–91.
19. Taylor DJ, Peterson AL, Pruiksma KE, et al. Internet and in-person cognitive behavioral therapy for insomnia in military personnel: a randomized clinical trial. Sleep 2017;40(6):zsx075.
20. de Bruin EJ, Bögels SM, Oort FJ, et al. Efficacy of cognitive behavioral therapy for insomnia in adolescents: a randomized controlled trial with internet therapy, group therapy and a waiting list condition. Sleep 2015;38(12):1913–26.
21. Blom K, Tarkian Tillgren H, Wiklund T, et al. Internet- vs. group-delivered cognitive behavior therapy for insomnia: a randomized controlled non-inferiority trial. Behav Res Ther 2015;70:47–55.
22. Holmqvist M, Vincent N, Walsh K. Web- vs. telehealth-based delivery of cognitive behavioral therapy for insomnia: a randomized controlled trial. Sleep Med 2014;15(2):187–95.
23. Thorndike FP, Ritterband LM, Gonder-Frederick LA, et al. A randomized controlled trial of an internet intervention for adults with insomnia: effects on co-morbid psychological and fatigue symptoms. J Clin Psychol 2013;69(10):1078–93.
24. Christensen H, Batterham PJ, Gosling JA, et al. Effectiveness of an online insomnia program (SHUTi) for prevention of depressive episodes (the

GoodNight Study): a randomised controlled trial. Lancet Psychiatry 2016;3(4):333–41.

25. Ye YY, Zhang YF, Chen J, et al. Internet-based cognitive behavioral therapy for insomnia (ICBT-i) improves comorbid anxiety and depression-a meta-analysis of randomized controlled trials. PLoS One 2015;10(11):e0142258.

26. Schubert JR, Arnedt JT. Management of insomnia in patients with alcohol use disorder. Curr Sleep Med Rep 2017;3(2):38–47.

27. Kuhn E, Weiss BJ, Taylor KL, et al. CBT-I coach: a description and clinician perceptions of a mobile app for cognitive behavioral therapy for insomnia. J Clin Sleep Med 2016;12(4):597–606.

28. Cheng P, Luik AI, Fellman-Couture C, et al. Efficacy of digital CBT for insomnia to reduce depression across demographic groups: a randomized trial. Psychol Med 2019;49(3):491–500.

29. McGrath ER, Espie CA, Power A, et al. Sleep to lower elevated blood pressure: a randomized controlled trial (SLEPT). Am J Hypertens 2017; 30(3):319–27.

30. Patel S, Ojo O, Genc G, et al. A computerized cognitive behavioral therapy randomized, controlled, pilot trial for insomnia in Parkinson's disease (ACCORD-PD study). J Clin Mov Disord 2017;4:16.

31. Jasper K, Weise C, Conrad I, et al. Internet-based guided self-help versus group cognitive behavioral therapy for chronic tinnitus: a randomized controlled trial. Psychother Psychosom 2014;83(4):234–46.

32. Weise C, Kleinstäuber M, Andersson G. Internet-delivered cognitive-behavior therapy for tinnitus: a randomized controlled trial. Psychosom Med 2016; 78(4):501–10.

33. Crawford MR, Espie CA, Luik AI, et al. Women with insomnia and debilitating migraines: sequential administration of online treatment- the Windsor study. Sleep 2017;40(suppl_1):A125.

34. Law E, Palermo T, Lord H, et al. Co-morbid pain and sleep disturbance: sleep outcomes in a randomized controlled trial of internet-based cognitive-behavioral therapy for insomnia. J Pain 2012;13(4):S97.

35. Zachariae R, Amidi A, Damholdt MF, et al. Internet-delivered cognitive-behavioral therapy for insomnia in breast cancer survivors: a randomized controlled trial. J Natl Cancer Inst 2018;110(8):880–7.

36. Ritterband LM, Bailey ET, Thorndike FP, et al. Initial evaluation of an Internet intervention to improve the sleep of cancer survivors with insomnia. Psychoon-cology 2012;21(7):695–705.

37. Bostock S, Luik AI, Espie CA. Sleep and productivity benefits of digital cognitive behavioral therapy for insomnia: a randomized controlled trial conducted in the workplace environment. J Occup Environ Med 2016;58(7):683–9.

38. Thiart H, Ebert DD, Lehr D, et al. Internet-based cognitive behavioral therapy for insomnia: a health economic evaluation. Sleep 2016;39(10):1769–78.

39. van der Zweerde T, Lancee J, Slottje P, et al. Cost-effectiveness of i-Sleep, a guided online CBT intervention, for patients with insomnia in general practice: protocol of a pragmatic randomized controlled trial. BMC Psychiatry 2016;16:85.

40. Espie CA, Kyle SD, Miller CB, et al. Attribution, cognition and psychopathology in persistent insomnia disorder: outcome and mediation analysis from a randomized placebo-controlled trial of online cognitive behavioural therapy. Sleep Med 2014; 15(8):913–7.

41. Lancee J, Eisma MC, van Straten A, et al. Sleep-related safety behaviors and dysfunctional beliefs mediate the efficacy of online CBT for insomnia: a randomized controlled trial. Cogn Behav Ther 2015;44(5):406–22.

42. Ho FY, Chung KF, Yeung WF, et al. Weekly brief phone support in self-help cognitive behavioral therapy for insomnia disorder: relevance to adherence and efficacy. Behav Res Ther 2014;63:147–56.

43. Ong JC, Kuo TF, Manber R. Who is at risk for dropout from group cognitive-behavior therapy for insomnia? J Psychosom Res 2008;64(4):419–25.

44. Edinger JD. Is it time to step up to stepped care with our cognitive-behavioral insomnia therapies? Sleep 2009;32(12):1539–41.

45. Espie CA. "Stepped care": a health technology solution for delivering cognitive behavioral therapy as a first line insomnia treatment. Sleep 2009;32(12): 1549–58.

46. Vincent N, Walsh K. Stepped care for insomnia: an evaluation of implementation in routine practice. J Clin Sleep Med 2013;9(3):227–34.

47. Thomas A, Grandner M, Nowakowski S, et al. Where are the behavioral sleep medicine providers and where are they needed? A geographic assessment. Behav Sleep Med 2016;14(6):687–98.

48. Internet/broadband fact sheet. Available at: http://www.pewinternet.org/fact-sheet/internet-broadband/. Accessed September 28, 2018.

49. Blom K, Jernelöv S, Lindefors N, et al. Facilitating and hindering factors in Internet-delivered treatment for insomnia and depression. Internet Interv 2016;4: 51–60.

50. Kaldo V, Jernelöv S, Blom K, et al. Guided internet cognitive behavioral therapy for insomnia compared to a control treatment – a randomized trial. Behav Res Ther 2015;71:90–100.

Moving?

Make sure your subscription moves with you!

To notify us of your new address, find your **Clinics Account Number** (located on your mailing label above your name), and contact customer service at:

Email: journalscustomerservice-usa@elsevier.com

800-654-2452 (subscribers in the U.S. & Canada)
314-447-8871 (subscribers outside of the U.S. & Canada)

Fax number: 314-447-8029

Elsevier Health Sciences Division
Subscription Customer Service
3251 Riverport Lane
Maryland Heights, MO 63043

*To ensure uninterrupted delivery of your subscription, please notify us at least 4 weeks in advance of move.

Printed and bound by CPI Group (UK) Ltd, Croydon, CR0 4YY

03/10/2024

01040370-0012